Going Against GMOs

The Fast-Growing Movement to Avoid

Unnatural Genetically Modified "Foods"

to Take Back Our Food and Health

by Melissa Diane Smith

For Martha and Larry —
So glad you're fighting
the good fight for our
community!
To pure food, good health,
& a healthy planet!
Love,
Melissa Diane Smith

Published by Melissa Diane Smith

Cover Design by Todd Engel of Engel Creative, Inc.
Cover Food Photos by iStock.com and Pornchai Mittongtare.
Author Photo by Deb Anderson of Vision Events Photography.

The purpose of this book is to provide general information for education and is not intended to be specific nutrition or medical advice for each person who reads it. Each person's health needs are unique. To obtain recommendations appropriate to your particular situation, please consult a qualified healthcare professional.

Every effort has been made to be accurate, but food formulations may change without notice. Always read labels carefully, and call specific companies when in doubt.

Neither the author nor the publisher is liable for any damages arising out of or in connection with the use of this book. This is a comprehensive limitation of liability that applies to all damages of any kind.

Printed in the United States of America on acid-free paper.

First Edition

This book is dedicated to the Earth

and the people and creatures

who live here.

Acknowledgments

Despite numerous challenges, I felt guided to write this book by many signs and people along the way.

My thanks go to the following individuals who helped give me key pieces of information or support during my research and writing: Mascha Miedaner; Rachel Linden; Shea Richland; Lesley McKeown; Cindy Bruwer; Alma Sychuk; Sigret and Keanne Thompson; Reza Shapouri; Ramiro Scavo; Kathy Iannacone; Kathleen Lohnes; Kimberly Knost; Kim Pebley; Sally Erroa; Stephanie St. Claire; Ann Loftfield; Mario Raso; Jazz Dolan; Bill McDorman; Belle Starr; Caroline Kinsman of the Non-GMO Project; Zack Kaldveer; James Palka; Ariane Glazer; Stacey Hall; Debbie Lee; Ron Smith; Bill Smith; Foster Gamble; Chris Anderson; and David Palmer.

Special thanks to my clients, most especially Marcia Popp not only for being a wonderful client and friend, but also a talented graphic artist and formatter, and to the many attendees at my presentations who helped me learn what was most pressing on people's minds through their questions. I also wish to extend my gratitude to the mothers, youngsters and pet owners who graciously shared their stories and tips with me: Lisa Sciandra; Kathleen Hallal of Moms Across America; Diana Reeves of GMO Free USA; Christina Le Beau; Rachel Parent of Kids Right to Know; Ginny Hensler; and songwriter Celia.

Kudos to Stacy Malkan and John and Ocean Robbins for planning and hosting excellent online summits that furthered my understanding of the many issues surrounding genetically modified foods.

My deep gratitude goes to the many experts I interviewed over the past several years, especially the following people who were generous with their time and information: Jeffrey Smith from the Institute for Responsible Technology; Andrew Kimbrell from the Center for Food

Safety; Michael Hansen, Ph.D., from Consumers Union; retired soil biologist and genetic engineer Thierry Vrain, Ph.D.; and integrative pediatrician Michelle Perro, M.D.

I am so appreciative of my loving family: Don, Ron, Rich, Marcia, Elena, and Michaela. Thanks also go to Mary Holden and Heather Karr who offered helpful editing suggestions; Paul Teitelbaum of Programs Plus, Inc.; Todd Engel of Engel Creative, Inc., for his book cover design; and Nancy Barnes of Stories To Tell who expertly guided me through many book production details. Finally, words cannot describe how grateful I am for the unwavering support of my dear friends Susan Hughes and Anne Kessell, and the friendship and excellent editing skills of Nicole Brechka and my mother Helen Smith. Each of these people encouraged me along the way, never letting me give up on my vision for this book and helping me see it through to completion. It is not an exaggeration to say that my mother, whose first name means "shining light" in Greek, was a guiding light through the whole process.

TABLE OF CONTENTS

SECTION 1: THE NON-GMO REVOLUTION THAT'S BREWING —AND THE REASONS FOR IT

SECTION 2: HOW TO GO AGAINST GMOs

SECTION 3: ADDITIONAL HELPFUL INFORMATION

Introduction

Let food be thy medicine, and medicine be thy food. – Hippocrates

When Hippocrates wrote those words more than 2,000 years ago, I'm sure he could not have fathomed that we would get to a time when some food wouldn't be *real food* anymore. He likely thought that life-giving food—all the living things that nature has bestowed on this earth to provide sustenance—would be constant and all we needed to do was find the right combination of foods on an individual basis to stay healthy. That's what I thought, too, first after experiencing the amazing power of the best foods on my own health in the early 1990s and then seeing how the right combination of real foods was the only answer for countless clients and readers of my books who had suffered from conditions ranging from diabetes to severe allergies.

In the past few decades when many of us focused on therapeutic diets to improve health, we were kept in the dark about something far more important: Many of our foods are no longer real food anymore. Multinational corporations changed our God- or nature-given foods on the *inside* in the most radical ways ever and our government allowed these food impostors known as genetically modified foods (or genetically engineered or genetically altered foods) to be secretly slipped into the food supply without our knowledge and without safety testing, starting in the mid to late 1990s. Though the U.S. Food and Drug Administration (FDA) dubbed genetically modified foods as "substantially equivalent" to regular foods, before that policy was put into place, the agency's own scientists warned that genetically modified foods were different and could lead to unexpected, hard-to-detect side effects that could adversely affect health, including new diseases, new allergens, new toxins, and nutritional problems.

In recent years growing numbers of people have learned this and more startling information that will be covered in this book, leaving them so concerned or so angry that many are now shopping defensively to avoid genetically modified foods. The changes in buying habits by individuals have built a collective and incredibly fast-growing food movement, which is changing business as usual in the food industry.

Many Americans want to learn more about genetically modified foods. Others still do not know basic facts that concern and often infuriate most who learn them. That's because the truth about genetically modified foods has been kept from the American public. It's time to shine a light on it from a consumer's point of view. That's what this book is all about.

Truth be told, I didn't originally want to write a book about genetically modified foods. I much prefer educating people about the healing power of real food. But circumstances in my journalistic and nutrition counseling work pushed me—almost forced me—to pay attention, learn much more about genetically modified food, and realize why this issue is so important for all of us to understand.

My Introduction into Genetically Modified Foods

I first learned about genetically modified foods in 2000 and 2001 when I was gathering information for my book *Going Against the Grain.* I turned on the news, heard about recalls of a type of genetically modified corn called StarLink corn that wasn't supposed to have entered our food supply but did, and saw reports of some people who said they had adverse reactions, including digestive trouble, skin reactions, and even anaphylactic shock, after eating corn-containing products from Taco Bell and other sources. I was concerned—horrified, really—and knew this was something I had to include in my book! I gathered up the limited information at the time to warn people about the potential dangers of genetically modified foods, explaining that StarLink corn was one of several types of pesticide-producing corn and that research in 1996 found that forcing a gene from one organism into the DNA of another can turn a nonallergenic food into an allergy-producing food.

Even the fundamental principles of genetically modifying foods bugged me. Pesticide could be in every cell of a type of corn? How crazy, I thought! Man splicing and dicing genes, the blueprint for life, and playing God with the foods the Earth naturally provided? How crazy, I thought! As a nutritionist, I knew that every time man has decided to artificially and dramatically alter natural foods—whether it was to create refined flours and sugars or refined or partially hydrogenated oils—it has ended up being to the detriment of public health.

I hoped people would stay away from genetically modified corn and soy after reading *Going Against the Grain*, but that didn't happen. Other information I covered in that book, like the fact that it's not only possible but common for people to react to gluten without having celiac disease, gradually seeped into the public consciousness. A gluten-free frenzy spread through the nation, but instead of eating more vegetables in place of grains—a central tenet of my book—most people who went gluten free began eating more highly processed, commercial gluten-free products that contained corn and soy. Not surprisingly, those gluten-free eaters never seemed to feel well. As a nutritionist, I knew that processed food products were unhealthy for us in many ways, but the factor I was increasingly wondering about was whether it was because they contained ingredients that were, in rapidly increasing amounts, genetically modified.

In 2010, I wrote *Gluten Free Throughout the Year* as a quick guide to steer busy people to more vegetables and to fewer processed foods and, yes, to fewer genetically modified gluten-free foods as well, even though I barely mentioned it. I also started delving into newer research on genetically modified (GM) foods to understand the topic better.

The more I pieced together new evidence starting to come out with basic information that had been kept from us about GM foods, the more disturbed I became. By that point, GM foods had infiltrated our food supply and were found in an estimated three-quarters of the foods sold in supermarkets, yet animal research (the only research available) linked

GM foods to immune system problems, gastrointestinal problems, infertility, accelerated aging, and more.

I was beginning to wonder when I counseled clients whether their symptoms and illnesses stemmed from an overly high-carbohydrate diet, a reaction to gluten or another food, or because of genetically modified foods. It was becoming impossible to tease out all of the variables. Right about then, I began providing nutritional coaching to Marcia, a client who had a huge impact on my thought processes.

MARCIA'S STORY

When Marcia, a 50-year-old graphic artist, began a nutrition coaching program with me in late 2010, she had numerous health problems, including multiple food and environmental allergies, and several heart-disease risk factors, including excess weight, high triglycerides, and low high-density lipoprotein (HDL) cholesterol (the "good" cholesterol). She also had been diagnosed in 1990 with a systemic immune condition known as Eosinophilia Myalgia Syndrome (EMS), which doctors thought she developed after taking a tainted batch of tryptophan supplements.

Marcia had already been following a gluten-free diet for eight years before she came to see me, in large part because she had read my previous book and felt better avoiding gluten. I advised a number of dietary changes to address her other food intolerances.

I knew that laboratory created genetically modified organisms (GMOs) were implicated in allergies and that the tryptophan linked to EMS had been produced using genetically modified bacteria,[1] so I recommended that she avoid all direct sources of GMOs in her diet to see if it made a difference. She was already avoiding wheat-based convenience foods that harbor hidden GMOs. So in her case, cutting out GMOs meant avoiding the soy-based edamame she had been eating because she thought it was "healthy," the aspartame-containing diet soda she often drank, and the corn-based ingredients that were hiding in her favorite gluten-free baked goods. I advised her to include more fresh vegetables (almost all of which aren't genetically modified) in her diet instead. I'm happy to say that it didn't take long for Marcia to see positive changes. Over several months, she and I were amazed at how avoiding genetically modified foods improved her health across the board.

What did avoiding GMOs do for Marcia's health? Consider these results:

- Within roughly a year, her seasonal allergies mostly disappeared.

- Working with her allergist, Marcia was able to stop all her allergy medications except for one she uses occasionally.

- Her body-wide inflammation subsided, her joints felt better, and her asthma symptoms improved so much that her lung function tests reached 98 percent—the highest they had ever been. (Now they're even higher at 105!)

- She lost 75 pounds and all of her heart-disease risk factors normalized.

- Just a few months after steering clear of GMOs, Marcia's immune cell counts (regularly tested to monitor her EMS condition) reached normal levels for the first time in almost 20 years! They have been consistent and normal ever since.

- In the first year of removing GM foods from her diet, Marcia cut her healthcare expenses by 50 percent and her dental expenses by 75 percent. She also saved $7,000 in medical expenses.

"Eliminating the GMOs has made the most impact for me," says Marcia. "The results have been amazing." Yes, I agree: the results were truly amazing!

How My Thinking and The Non-GMO Movement Evolved

Marcia's experience had me wondering whether *any* therapeutic diet could resolve people's health problems or keep them healthy if they were having reactions like Marcia did to even a few genetically modified foods. I wished food was still good, old-fashioned *food* so I could just focus on therapeutic diets. But I had to face the fact that that was no longer the case. Genetically modified food had become the food issue of our time.

I needed to understand the topic far better, so I delved into learning everything I could about GMOs. I interviewed food safety experts; attended conferences and listened to numerous webinars, telesummits, and online conferences; and talked with farmers, sustainable food advocates, physicians, nutrition professionals, and consumers, learning the types of questions people asked over and over again. I also studied independent research—in other words, research not affiliated in any way with the biotechnology industry that develops and markets genetically modified foods.

I discovered that far more had been hidden from the American public than I realized. In a nutshell, we had never been given any upfront information about GM foods and therefore, had never had the opportunity to discuss whether or not we wanted them in our food. Instead, because of a policy the United States developed that was out of step with the majority of countries in the world, GM foods had been secretly pushed into our food supply without our knowledge, making us all uninformed participants— or guinea pigs—in a massive feeding experiment.

What's more, when I sifted through the hype and really studied the evidence, there was no good reason for consumers to eat them. I firmly believe that the genetic engineering of our foods would never have gone so far if the public had been given straight information from the start, including warnings issued by the FDA's own scientists and other people and organizations.

As a nutritionist, health journalist, and concerned citizen, I couldn't really sit on this information. I began writing about the topic on my blog and speaking about it in my community.

From 2011 to 2013, I was researching, interviewing, studying non-GMO foods on the market, writing, speaking, and counseling new clients, wrapping my mind around every aspect of the GMO issue. As I was getting up to speed on information about GM foods, more Americans were learning bits and pieces of information from friends or social media, not liking what they learned, and becoming increasingly upset as new GM foods were green-lighted into the food system despite widespread public disapproval.

Though many Americans still knew nothing about this fundamental change in their food, those who were aware of the situation were getting fed up with genetically modified foods literally being shoved down their throats without their knowledge or consent. They began taking their power back by learning where GMOs are hidden and not buying foods that contained them. In the last year especially, food companies have been taking notice of this fast-growing non-GMO movement and responding, making major business changes based on growing consumer demand. As a journalist, I saw this as a big story, but I also thought that it wasn't being covered in a way that Americans needed to hear or could understand.

When counseling clients, I saw that those who were attempting to eliminate GMOs from their diets were making nutritional mistakes, either by eating hidden sources of genetically modified foods without realizing it or eating non-GMO "junk food" that set them up for other health problems. I have counseled people on many types of diets, and no matter what diet someone eats, there's one constant: most individuals are getting large amounts of GMOs from grain- and sugar-based processed convenience foods they're eating. The easiest way to teach people to automatically cut the top GMOs out of their diets in a healthy way is to have them ditch processed foods and substitute more fresh vegetables and fruits, which generally aren't genetically modified. To go against

GMOs, individuals have to go against the grain of what most people in the United States are eating. That subject is my specialty.

A New Kind of Going Against the Grain

As you read this book, keep in mind that eating non-GMO and organic foods isn't a radical new diet. It isn't about people being "fussy" about their food. It simply means eating food the way nature intended.

Twenty years ago all our food was non-GMO—produced without laboratory created genetically modified organisms. Seventy-five years ago, all our food was organic—in other words, produced without synthetic fertilizers and pesticides. There's a meme circulating on the Internet, which in a few simple words summarizes this point. It says: Try organic food ... or as your grandparents called it, *"Food."*

When it comes to easily being able to eat organic, non-GMO food, I'm well aware that the system is stacked against us, and it's particularly stacked against the poor. Government subsidies—in other words, our taxpayer dollars—go to support "farmers," mainly large corporations that produce foods like wheat, corn and soy on a massive scale that we don't need. Then various forms of those ingredients are added to processed foods and used to unhealthfully fatten up animals. Vegetable and fruit growers, and organic food growers, which we desperately need, are offered little or no financial support.[2][3] It's a messed-up, unhealthy food system.

That means it's all the more important for those of us who can eat real food to do so. If enough of us do this, it will change the system and make it possible for all of us to affordably eat real food again. I certainly never thought we'd have to fight for the right to eat real food. But that's the situation we are in now. I consider it a patriotic duty to go against GMOs and fight for a better food system.

WHAT YOU'LL LEARN IN THIS BOOK

From many different fronts, the message has been getting louder and louder about the need for a consumer-friendly guide about the fast-growing non-GMO food movement, the reasons for it, and steps for removing genetically modified foods from the diet in a healthy way. I heard the call. Just as I felt guided 12 years ago to reveal critical information that had been kept from us about grains, I now feel compelled to disclose important basics that have been kept from us about genetically modified foods and the radically different agricultural system that goes with them—information we all should have been told decades ago.

In Chapter 1, I will reveal how quickly the non-GMO movement is growing and how it is prompting large and small businesses to make changes in the foods they offer. In Chapters 2 through 4, I'll run down the compelling reasons why so many consumers now want to go against GMOs.

In Section 2, I'll put on my nutritionist hat to provide comprehensive advice about how to avoid GMOs, offering practical guidelines, tips, shopping and eating out suggestions, as well as easy recipes for people on many different diets. I end the book with Section 3, which provides additional helpful information, including appendices and resources.

Whether you have been wondering about GMOs, never heard about them before, or want to avoid them but don't know how, do yourself a favor and dig into this book. I'm confident you'll get the complete rundown on the current state of our food system and how we all can individually and collectively get back to real food to once again make it our best medicine.

SECTION 1:

The Non-GMO Revolution That's Brewing —and the Reasons for It

Chapter 1:

The Fast-Growing Food Movement
That's Shaking Up the Food Industry

The movement to avoid laboratory created, genetically modified organisms (GMOs) hidden in foods is growing so swiftly and with such force that it's becoming a revolution. It was *the* absolute fastest-growing food movement in the natural foods industry in 2013, and as you'll learn in this chapter, it's shaking up the food world.

You won't hear about this movement on the nightly news. It's rarely covered by the mainstream media. It is a grassroots movement that has taken place under the radar and it has spread mostly through word of mouth, social media, and community-oriented educational events. But the passion about this type of eating by growing numbers of people is so strong, it is changing business as usual, causing many food manufacturers and some grocery store and restaurant chains to make major changes in the foods they offer.

GMOs are defined as organisms in which the genetic material (DNA) has been altered in a way that does not occur in nature by using genetic engineering techniques. Genetically modified (GM) foods are "foods" produced from those novel organisms. The non-GMO food movement means that people are now insisting on eating pure, unadulterated food as nature intended, not the newfangled creations.

THE GROWING DEMAND FOR NON-GMO FOODS

The U.S. Food and Drug Administration says genetically altered foods are safe and not fundamentally different than the *real* animal and plant foods people have always eaten; however, increasing numbers of individuals don't accept those statements or don't want to take unnecessary chances eating GM foods. Ten years ago, most Americans *said* they would avoid

GMOs if labeled. Now millions are no longer waiting. The more people learn about GMOs and how they were introduced into our food supply without transparency, the more they don't like them and are moving away from them. *Fortunately, we now have the ability to avoid GMOs with or without mandatory federal labeling.*

One of the key ways to avoid foods with GM ingredients is to seek out products with a Non-GMO Project Verified seal. The Non-GMO Project was started by retailers who believed that consumers in North America should have access to clearly labeled non-GMO food and products. It's North America's only independent verification program for products made according to the best practices for GMO avoidance, including testing of at-risk ingredients.

Sales of Non-GMO Project Verified products skyrocketed from $0 in 2010 when the label launched to more than $3.5 billion just three years later.[4] Non-GMO products are in such demand that there are now more than 15,000 verified products, and sales of products that qualify for a Non-GMO verification enjoy a sales spike between 15 to 30 percent.[5][6]

Projections are that this is the beginning of a huge buying trend. Market research publisher *Packaged Facts* estimates that by 2017 non-GMO products will make up around 30 percent of total food and beverage sales, with a value of about $264 billion.[7]

USDA certified organic products cannot intentionally include any GM ingredients and their sales also have increased. In 2012, there was a 12 percent increase in sales of organic products, and Organic Trade Association surveys show that 22 percent of the respondents now cite avoiding GMOs as a primary reason to eat organic food, up from 17 percent in 2011.[8][9]

Non-GMO and organic products have become so big in the marketplace, they account for a significant portion of the products in the aisles of most natural food stores today, and they're starting to find shelf space in conventional grocery stores, too. Small food companies in communities across the country also are beginning to make business changes in response to strong consumer demand for non-GMO products and restaurant items. A few examples from my own community: just in the past two years, a local movie theater started selling non-GMO popcorn popped in non-GMO canola oil; a tamale company is now using non-GMO corn masa and non-GMO organic safflower oil in its tamales; and a few farm-to-table restaurants made changes in some of their ingredients. One vegetarian restaurant took GMOs out of almost all of the foods on its menu!

CONSUMER COMMENTS DRIVING CHANGES IN FOOD

Not only are more people shopping non-GMO, they're speaking up loudly and en masse telling companies they don't want GM ingredients in their foods. After a 2012 study by the Cornucopia Institute, an organic and agriculture policy group, found that certain brands of cereal contained GM ingredients, some natural food stores pulled those cereals off their shelves.[10] Consumers responded with a flurry of angry website and Facebook comments to the companies whose cereals were found to contain GMOs.[11] The public outcry prompted one of the companies, Kashi, to pledge that beginning in 2015, all new foods it introduces will be Non-GMO Project Verified and will contain at least 70 percent USDA certified organic ingredients.[12]

General Mills also felt the squeeze of consumer pressure against its iconic cereal Cheerios. In 2013, customers flooded the Cheerios Facebook page with comments demanding the company stop using GMOs. At the beginning of 2014, the company responded, announcing it would be manufacturing its original Cheerios breakfast cereal without GM ingredients, swapping out the cornstarch and sugar in its cereal for non-GMO versions.[13][14]

Post Foods followed suit just days later, announcing it slightly revamped its Original Grape-Nuts cereal to remove the GM ingredients—and it went through third party verification to receive the Non-GMO Project Verified seal. Post said it is listening to customers and exploring the possibilities of having more of its cereals become non-GMO verified.[15][16]

*The same food companies that offer non-GMO versions of their foods
in the European Union, where protest against GMOs has been high, use
GMOs in the North American versions. The United States and Canada
are two of the few countries where GM foods aren't labeled.* Those facts
have fired up North American consumers all the more.

The numbers of people choosing to shop and eat non-GMO have swelled
to such a point that the largest natural foods retailer, Whole Foods Market,
responded to repeated customer requests for more non-GMO options.
In March 2013, Whole Foods announced it would require labeling of
GM foods sold in its stores for products that were either not organic or
not verified by the Non-GMO Project by 2018. The move gave their
supplier partners five years to source non-GMO ingredients or clearly
label products as containing GMOs.[17] As a result, many food companies
that work with Whole Foods are now seeking non-GMO ingredients.

Non-GMO awareness and activism also have extended into the streets.
In April and May 2013, with the help of Facebook, people around the
country and world organized the unprecedented worldwide March
Against Monsanto, in which 2 million people around the globe marched
against GMOs. A few days later, on May 27, 2013, *The New York Times*
ran the article "Seeking Food Ingredients That Aren't Gene-Altered,"
with the lead paragraph stating: *Food companies big and small are
struggling to replace genetically modified ingredients with conventional
ones.*[18]

Restaurants Making Changes

Restaurants, especially smaller, locally owned, farm-to-table restaurants,
also are gradually making changes. I educated five forward-thinking
restaurant owners in Tucson in 2011 and 2012, taught them how to avoid
GMOs in meal preparation, and worked with them to offer special Non-
GMO Pure Food Dinners. All the dinners were incredibly popular and
well attended, with more than 25 people at every single one.

In March 2013, the national chain Chipotle Mexican Grill, Inc., took major action toward becoming non-GMO. Known for its "food with integrity" message, with more than 1,500 restaurants nationwide, Chipotle became the first U.S. company to post labels on its website to let customers know which of its menu items contained GMO ingredients and it committed to phasing out the use of GM ingredients as quickly as possible.[19]

WALL STREET RESPONDING TO THE NON-GMO TRENDS

On the Friday following Chipotle's announcement in October 2013, Chipotle's stock soared 15 percent to an all-time high.[20] Financial investors are also taking note of the growing negative sentiment toward GMOs and GM seed companies such as Monsanto. Financial website *Insider Monkey* reported in 2013:

> Monsanto Company has had one of the most up-and-down years of the stocks we track. Shares of the ag behemoth (Monsanto) have been unable to get on a run in 2013, as constant drama over GMOs seems to be hitting the newswires daily. With that in mind, it appears that some hedge funds want nothing to do with it.[21]

Jeffrey Vinik's Vinik Asset Management and Sean Cullinan's fund, Point State Capital, dropped close to $100.8 million worth and about $54.7 million worth, respectively, of their Monsanto stock.

OPERATION MONSANTO STOCK PLUNGE

In April 2014, the food activist groups Organic Spies and Food Democracy Now launched a campaign named Operation Monsanto Stock Plunge that urged investors to sell shares of biotech companies like Monsanto. The campaign particularly encouraged people to sell Fidelity, Vanguard and State Street mutual funds that own and control enormous volumes of Monsanto stock.

A petition on the Food Democracy Now website states that Monsanto "has cornered a monopoly on genetically engineering the food that we eat to either be tolerant of the weed killer Roundup or to contain (an) insecticidal gene. ... As Monsanto continues to lead the fight against GMO labeling in the U.S. with deceptive PR and ad campaigns, it's time to remind them that corrupting our democracy to protect their profits has a price."[22]

Less than a day after the launch of Operation Monsanto Stock Plunge, Monsanto stocks fell steadily all day long. Nasdaq, which is weighted heavily toward technology and biotechnology companies, had its worse day since November 2011, meaning mutual fund holders likely helped cause the plunge and directly influenced the movement of billions of dollars on Wall Street.[23]

A Food Movement That Isn't Going Away

Consumers are starting to realize the incredible power they have. They're paying much more attention to where their food comes from than they did even 10 years ago. They are concerned about several artificial, corporate-driven ingredients, but GMOs are quickly reaching the top of many people's lists. Food companies, restaurants, and Wall Street in turn are all starting to pay attention. Food manufacturers and restaurants are scrambling to adapt to this burgeoning consumer demand and secure sources of non-GMO ingredients, and investors are noticing the trends and rewarding companies that are meeting the demand.

As you'll learn in the next few chapters, there are wide-ranging reasons for the non-GMO food movement. Every indication is that the movement will continue to grow in popularity among people from different demographics—from those concerned about protecting the environment to people worried about chemical-laden industrial agriculture to people on various diets. Unlike food movements that favor one type of eating, such as people who eat gluten free, eating non-GMO attracts people from all different types of food disciplines, from those on the Standard

American Diet to those on therapeutic or specialty diets ranging from high-protein/low carb to vegan.

For example, a 2013 *Gluten-Free Living* website survey found that the majority of respondents said they now avoid GMOs in addition to avoiding foods that contain gluten. Nearly half of the respondents—47 percent—said it was "very important" to avoid GMOs and they only buy non-GMO gluten-free products. Another 36 percent said avoiding GMOs was "somewhat important" and they buy non-GMO gluten-free products when possible.[24]

Uneasiness about eating genetically modified foods is steadily growing in mainstream America as well. A 2013 *New York Times* poll showed that three-quarters of Americans expressed concern about GMOs in their food, with most of them worried about the effects on people's health.[25]

A separate survey by The NPD Group, a leading global information company, found that more than half of U.S. consumers say they are concerned about genetically modified foods, up from 43 percent in 2002. Levels of apprehension have risen as well. Less than 10 percent of adults were "very" or "extremely" worried about GMOs in 2002, but now that concern level is at more than 20 percent of adults, and has steadily increased, according to NPD's Food Safety Monitor, which continually tracks consumer awareness and concern about food safety issues and eating intentions.[26]

In addition, while more than half of U.S. consumers are apprehensive about GMOs, many still think GMOs have some benefits. As you'll read in the next chapter, GMOs offer no benefits to consumers!

To understand the many reasons for public concern and the growing shift toward non-GMO in the marketplace, it's important to learn some basics. The next chapter will give you a crash course on GMOs from a consumer's point of view, helping you understand why growing numbers of shoppers are saying no to GMOs and are committed to buying and eating non-GMO long term.

Chapter 2:

GMOs: The Food Issue of Our Time

Imagine engineers manipulating the seeds of common food crops to make plants that produce their own insecticide or that are resistant to chemical herbicides that kill other plants. These sound like scenarios that you might see in a scary futuristic sci-fi movie, yet they happen routinely today and most of us are unknowingly eating foods that are genetically modified in one of these ways—or both of them—every day.

Now stretch your mind further and visualize seeds of those crops being patented and owned by the world's largest chemical companies, and farmers being sued if the wind happens to blow seeds or pollen from those man-made plants and they take root in farmers' fields—even if farmers had no desire to grow those altered plants. Picture the powers-that-be in our country saying that these modified plants are essentially the same as traditional foods so these high-tech, industry-tinkered "foods" don't have to be labeled, yet they are so different that they can be patented. And corporations can make millions off them and keep buying more seeds and altering them to control an increasing percentage of the world's food and seed supply.

Does this sound completely outrageous and far-fetched? Well, there's no need to think of it as fiction. Everything described here is exactly what has happened in our food system. It's our current food reality.

As unimaginable as the scenario described above may seem, growing numbers of Americans are learning bits and pieces of the cold hard truth about what has secretly been done to our food system. Essentially, we are the first generation to have newfangled, untested genetically modified organisms (GMOs) imperceptibly, yet pervasively, hidden in our foods.

THE FDA POLICY ON GM FOODS

The official U.S. Food and Drug Administration (FDA) policy on GM foods from 1992 states: *"The agency is not aware of any information showing that foods derived by these new methods differ from other foods in any meaningful or uniform way...."*

More than 44,000 pages of internal records made public due to a lawsuit seven years later revealed that wasn't true. Before the policy was announced, the FDA's own scientists repeatedly warned that genetically modified foods could lead to unexpected, hard-to-detect side effects, including new diseases, new allergens, new toxins, and nutritional problems, and should require long-term safety studies.[27]

THE VERY DIFFERENT U.S. POLICY ON GMOs

Ninety percent of Americans, which includes an almost even split of support among Democrats, Republicans, and Independents, want genetically modified foods at least labeled.[28] [29] But the United States is one of the few countries in which GM foods are not labeled or banned. There's more than meets the eye to even that: You see, the FDA's own scientists urged their superiors to require safety studies on GMOs, but their concerns were kept secret and weren't acted upon. Instead, genetically modified foods were fast-tracked onto the market without safety tests.[30]

On May 29, 1992, as part of a deregulatory initiative, Vice President Dan Quayle announced the U.S. policy that genetically engineered crops are "substantially equivalent" to regular crops and therefore do not need to be labeled or tested before being put on the market. One conference on GMOs described it as a policy based on politics, not science![31]

Consequently, contrary to what most people believe, the FDA has never approved a GM food as safe. The organization actually does not carry out safety tests on GM foods.

Instead, the FDA operates a voluntary program for pre-market review of GM foods. After that review, the FDA acknowledges that, based on the research provided by the company seeking to commercialize the GM foods, the manufacturer has concluded that the GM products are safe.[32] [33] [34] If the company claims that its foods are safe, the FDA accepts those conclusions with no further questions.[35]

This policy, which still stands today, is the reason why GM crops were slipped into the U.S. food system without mandatory testing or labeling and without the public's knowledge or consent. Canada, which has mostly acted in accordance with U.S. policy, also has this same lack of transparency about the presence of GMOs in its food system.[36]

Most other countries, on the other hand, agree that genetically modified foods are different than traditional foods, have different risks, and therefore require regulation. At least 26 countries, including Russia, Switzerland, Australia, China, India, France, Germany, Hungary, Luxembourg, Greece, Bulgaria, Poland, Italy, and Mexico, have total or partial bans on GMOs, and Europe has 174 GMO-free zones. More than 60 countries have significant restrictions on the production or sale of GMOs and require labeling of GM foods so consumers can make informed decisions about their food.[37]

The actions the United States took have led us to purchase GM foods for decades without realizing it, entirely by accident, because we were kept in the dark about what we were buying. GMOs are estimated to be in 75 to 80 percent of the foods sold today in U.S. supermarkets; comparatively, GMOs are estimated to be in single-digit percentages of the foods sold in stores in the European Union.

As Americans learn this and other convoluted, less-than-ethical details about untested GM foods in our food supply, the angrier they get. But there's even more. Many basic facts about GMOs simply don't sit well with most who learn about them.

What Are GMOs?

Genetically modified organisms (GMOs) are organisms whose DNA has been altered using genetic engineering to confer different traits. In technical terms, genes from the DNA of one species are extracted and forced into the DNA of an unrelated plant or animal typically by using bacteria or viruses to "infect" animal or plant cells with the new DNA or by shooting cells with a "gene gun."

If a GMO is used for food, that product is called a genetically modified (GM) food. In everyday language, though, the terms GMO and GM food are used interchangeably to mean a "food" produced using GMOs.

GM foods look exactly the same as traditional foods but they're very different on the inside.

BASICS ABOUT GMOs

Unlike food that has been grown from seeds handed down through generations, genetically modified foods are created in laboratories. Genetic engineers artificially insert genes from bacteria, viruses, or animals into the DNA of a food crop or animal to make a genetically modified organism that would never occur in nature, to confer new traits.

Many people think genetically engineered crops are like those that are naturally bred, but that's not true. Natural breeding only takes place between closely related forms of life, such as pigs with pigs or wheat with wheat. Genetic engineering involves transferring genes across species that could not mate. In order to breach species barriers set up by nature and force the foreign DNA into the unrelated species, genetic engineers use a variety of methods, including using viruses or bacteria to "infect" animal or plant cells with the new DNA, or coating DNA onto tiny metal pellets and firing it with a special gun into the cells.

There is global agreement that genetic engineering is different than conventional breeding, and that safety assessments should be completed for all GM foods before they are allowed on the market.

The United States, however, unlike all other developed countries, does not require safety testing for GM plants. The FDA makes no conclusions about the safety of GM food, but says it is up to the companies to determine safety of any GM food.

– Michael Hansen, Ph.D., Senior Scientist at Consumers Union, the public policy arm of Consumer Reports, who has testified at many government hearings on the topic

Actually, it's not just one gene that is inserted. A whole new gene package known as a "gene construct" is used—not only the foreign gene to try to create a new trait, but also promoter genes to turn the new gene on and suppressor genes to turn the gene off. In most of the GM crops currently on the market, engineers also typically have attached an antibiotic-resistance marker gene to the foreign gene so they can determine which of the thousands of cells they shot have the foreign gene in their DNA. (For those interested in the technical details: Engineers put all the cells they shoot in a Petri dish that contains the antibiotic. The cells that survive are resistant to the antibiotic, which means they are also the ones that contain the foreign gene.)

What this means to you and me is that many foods today look the same as they used to look before GMOs. They may even taste the same. But on the inside, they're very different, with foreign genes forced into the most fundamental inner workings of plants or animals to confer new traits in a Frankenstein-like way. This is a key reason why Europeans often call genetically modified foods "Frankenfoods."

THE BIG FIVE

Most genetically modified ingredients are derived from the top five genetically modified crops grown in the United States listed below. The five crops are overwhelmingly genetically modified to be herbicide tolerant—in other words, to tolerate repeated spraying of herbicide that kills other plants. Corn and cotton are also often genetically modified to produce their own internal pesticide, and soy may soon be added to that list.

Corn   Soy

Cotton (found in foods such as   Sugar Beets (found in beet sugar or
         cottonseed oil)   most foods that contain "sugar")

Canola (found in foods such as
         canola oil)

Here's another key fact to know: Almost all of the genetically modified foods on the market are what I call "pesticide plants" or "toxic chemical plants," genetically altered to either produce their own chemical insecticide inside every cell or to tolerate lots of chemical herbicide, such as Roundup weed killer. (The latter are known as "Roundup Ready" plants. They don't die from being sprayed with Roundup but everything else around them does.)

Virtually all of the top five genetically modified crops in the U.S.—sugar beets, soy, corn, canola (as in canola oil), and cotton (as in cottonseed oil)—are genetically modified to be herbicide tolerant, which means lots of extra herbicide is being sprayed on the outside of the plant. (It's important to know that the herbicide readily moves into all parts of a plant and doesn't just stay on the outside.) In addition, many types of corn today produce their own insecticide inside every cell, and most often, corn is "stacked" to have both traits: herbicide tolerance as well as the internal insecticide.

CLAIMS ABOUT GMOS REFUTED BY RESEARCH

Biotech companies, such as the largest GM seed company Monsanto, claim that genetically modified crops use less pesticide and increase crop yields, with the ultimate goal being to "help feed the world." Many of us have heard those statements in mainstream stories on TV or read them in newspapers such as *The New York Times* that most of us assume they must be accurate. Research, however, shows a different story.

Though biotech companies said growing GM crops would lead to less pesticide use, research shows that GMOs have actually led to increased herbicide use. Spraying of crops with herbicides such as glyphosate, the active ingredient in Roundup, has led to the development and spread of so-called "superweeds"—weeds that adapt to and withstand glyphosate, resulting in yet more spraying.[38] How much additional herbicide is being used? It's hard to believe, but *527 million more pounds of herbicides were used on GM herbicide-tolerant corn, cotton, and soy between 1996 and 2011, the first 16 years of genetically modified crops being used,* according to a 2012 report published in *Environmental Sciences Europe.*[39]

The biotech companies' proposed solution to the development of superweeds is to create new GM crops resistant to more toxic herbicides, such as 2,4-D, a major component of Agent Orange, the Vietnam War defoliant.[40][41] If new genetically engineered forms of corn and soybeans tolerant of 2,4-D are allowed on the market, the volume of 2,4-D sprayed could drive herbicide usage upward by another 50 percent.[42] Opponents say developing new herbicide-resistant crops isn't a solution to the problem of superweeds: Weeds would simply adapt and become resistant to any herbicides that are used in large amounts.

Just as many weeds have adapted to the herbicides that are used on GM herbicide-resistant crops, many insects have adapted to the insecticide (known as Bt for *Bacillus thuringiensis*) that is in pesticide-producing GM corn and cotton crops. Insects are now munching away on the corn and cotton without consequences, creating a growing number of hard-to-kill "super insects." As of 2010, five of 13 major insect species had become largely immune to the Bt poisons in GMO corn and cotton, compared to just one species in 2005, say scientists in a 2013 paper from the journal *Nature Biotechnology*.[43] Pest adaptation makes the built-in GM pesticide less effective over time, prompting farmers to revert to spraying chemical pesticides after just a few years.[44] [45]

SUPERWEEDS, SUPER INSECTS, AND THE PESTICIDE TREADMILL

Almost all of the genetically modified crops grown are herbicide resistant or pesticide producing. Their use has led to the development of:

- **"Superweeds"** that have become resistant to the herbicides sprayed on them;

- **"Super insects"** that have largely become immune to the built-in pesticide;

- **"A pesticide treadmill,"** in which farmers get caught in a situation where they are forced to spray more and more—and increasingly toxic—chemicals to control insect and weed populations that continue to develop resistance to each new type or class of pesticides.

The Pesticide Action Network calls the development of "superweeds" and "super insects" classic cases of the "pesticide treadmill," also called the "pesticide trap." Farmers get caught on the treadmill as they are forced to use more and more—and increasingly toxic—chemicals to control insects and weeds that develop resistance to pesticides.[46]

Furthermore, GMOs do not, on average, increase crop yields, according to a 2009 report entitled "Failure to Yield" by Doug Gurian-Sherman, Ph.D., Senior Scientist at the Union of Concerned Scientists and former biotech adviser to the U.S. Environmental Protection Agency.[47] According to the report:

- Herbicide-tolerant GM corn and soy don't increase yields any more than conventional.

- Non-GM plant breeding and farming methods increase yields far more.

- "Traditional breeding outperforms genetic engineering hands down," wrote Gurian-Sherman.

Other research suggests that GM soybeans give consistently lower yields than their non-GM counterparts, and that 50 percent of this reduction may be due to the disruption in genes caused by the GM transformation process.[48]

A study published in the peer-reviewed *International Journal of Agricultural Sustainability* in 2013 analyzed data on agricultural productivity in North America and western Europe over the past 50 years: Researchers found that genetic engineering used in North American staple crop production is lowering yields and increasing pesticide use compared to western Europe.[49] On the *Sustainable Pulse* website, the lead author of the study, University of Canterbury professor Jack Heinemann, Ph.D., wrote: "Europe has learned to grow more food per hectare and use fewer chemicals in the process. The American choices in biotechnology are causing it to fall behind Europe in productivity and sustainability."[50]

No Benefits for Consumers

The next logical question is what, then, do genetically modified foods do for us, the consumers who have been unknowingly eating them? The answer is nothing beneficial. As surprising as that answer is to most people, that's the truth. Take it from Andrew Kimbrell, the Executive Director of the Center for Food Safety and an environmental lawyer who has been studying GMOs for 25 years. He sums up the lack of benefits from GMOs for consumers this way:

> The dirty secret of the biotech companies is after 30 years and hundreds of billions of dollars of public and private investment, they have yet to produce anything that benefits the consumer. There's no better taste, no better nutrition, no lower price—in other words, zero benefits and potential risks. That's the dirty little secret that is hardly ever reported.
>
> No one wakes up in the morning saying they want to buy a genetically modified food. That's why those companies don't want GM foods labeled. The biotech companies don't want the consumer to be able to have the choice to say, "I want the same price, less risky version."[51]

[With genetically modified foods]... there's no better taste, no better nutrition, no lower price—in other words, zero benefits and potential risks.

– Andrew Kimbrell, Executive Director of the Center for Food Safety

Corporations the Beneficiaries of GMOs

So, if GMOs don't do anything helpful for us, who, then, actually benefits from GMOs? The answer to that question is the chemical companies producing these patented GM seeds and their matching herbicides.

"This is about chemical companies selling more of their chemicals," says Kimbrell, who is also the author of *Your Right to Know: Genetic Engineering and the Secret Changes in Your Food.*

Yes, that's right, over the past few decades, agrichemical corporations, such as Monsanto, DuPont, and Syngenta, have increasingly been buying the seeds from which our plant foods are grown, genetically modifying them for their benefit, patenting those new creations, and making an outrageous amount of money locking farmers into regularly buying the patented seeds and herbicides, often at inflated prices.

The Issue of Patenting Seeds

One of the most controversial aspects surrounding genetic engineering is the patenting of seeds. For most of history, the U.S. Patent and Trademark Office did not allow for the patenting of life. But that changed in 1980 when the U.S. Supreme Court ruled five to four that a live, human-made microorganism—in the case being tried, a bacterium invented by General Electric to clean up oil spills—could be patented. Ironically, that bacterium was never used. However, agrichemical corporations seized the opportunity to use this ruling to their advantage, acquiring patents on hundreds of seeds for key food crops, and thereby snatching never-before-seen control and monopoly of our food.[52]

What this means is that if you're a farmer who wants to grow GM crops, you must buy seeds (and the herbicides that go with them) from biotech companies every year instead of using seeds saved from each year's crop (something farmers had done for millennia). But it gets outrageously more disadvantageous for farmers: GM crops are not grown in enclosed, contained areas but out in the open where their pollen or seeds can easily spread and contaminate non-GMO crops. So if you're a farmer who opts out of growing GM crops, but happens to get some patented GM crops accidentally growing on your land because wind, rain, or birds brought GM pollen or seeds to your property, biotech companies can actually take you to court saying that you violated the law by using their patented seeds and demanding payment for their use. Since 1997, Monsanto has filed suit against farmers 145 times in the United States, according to the company's website.[53] Farmers have come together to fight this unfair practice. However, the courts have not yet ruled on their side to change this situation.[54]

Patenting seeds also means that a select few companies own an increasing percentage of our food. A 2008 report entitled "Who Owns Nature?" on corporate concentration in commercial food and farming revealed these startling numbers:[55] [56]

- The top 10 seed companies account for $14,785 million—or two-thirds (67%)—of the global proprietary seed market.

- The world's largest seed company, Monsanto, owns almost one-quarter (23%) of the world's proprietary seeds.

- The top three companies (Monsanto, DuPont, Syngenta) together account for $10,282 million, or 47%, of the worldwide proprietary seed market.

FOOD INTEGRITY AND FOOD SECURITY ISSUES

The situation that has developed from the use of GMOs, the practice of patenting of GMOs, and the fact that only a handful of corporations control so many seeds and cash crops, threatens our food safety and security in many ways. First consider the contamination issue. GMOs are unnatural life forms. Once released into the environment, GMOs cannot be cleaned up or recalled. Unlike chemical and nuclear contamination, which can be contained in many cases, genetic pollution cannot be isolated and separated from the environment it's in. This means that maintaining the purity or integrity of organic and heirloom (also called "heritage") varieties of crops that are related to common GM crops is becoming increasingly difficult, if not impossible, in areas where GM crops are grown.

Also, seed was formerly a free, renewable resource, but as corporations have patented and privatized seed, it has become a costly, non-renewable farm input for the farmers. Control of seed, therefore, has moved away from farmers and local communities to large corporations, threatening food security around the globe.

As more farmers repeatedly grow the same variety of GM seed, other heirloom seeds are in danger of becoming extinct. These seeds hold the genetic diversity that could offer traits to ward off diseases and better adapt to climate changes in the future, making them critical for our long-term food security.

AN EXTENSION OF INDUSTRIAL AGRICULTURE

If you stop and think about it, the use of GMOs is an extension or furthering of chemical-based industrial agriculture. At its core, industrial agriculture focuses not only on the heavy use of synthetic fertilizers and pesticides but also on *monoculture*—the practice of growing single crops, such as corn, soy, and wheat, intensively on a large scale. The overproduction of single crops like these—crops we don't need—means they end up being used as feed for factory-farmed animals for meat and added in large amounts to processed foods, which are unhealthy foods that should be avoided.[57]

Monocultures, upon which the GM agriculture system is based, can lead to the spread of pests and diseases. A uniform crop also is susceptible to a pathogen. For example, if there's a blight or an issue with pests or fungus that spreads through that one crop, the crop can die and lead to an extreme food shortage. This happened during Ireland's Great Potato Famine in 1845-1849. While GMOs were not to blame back then, a monoculture agriculture system was. Ireland's food crisis started with heavy reliance on just one or two varieties of potato. Then, a blight spread through Irish potato crops, resulting in them failing in consecutive years and more than a million people dying from starvation or famine-related diseases.[58] The same type of situation could develop in a GMO-based single-crop-focused agriculture system.

The real answer to food secure agriculture is a diversity of locally produced crops, which makes a food system resilient to a variety of weather, soil, and environmental conditions. If one crop fails, others will survive and help fill in the gap.

THE GMO AGRICULTURE SYSTEM

- **An extension of chemical-based industrial agriculture**

- **Emphasizes use of pesticides, such as insecticides and herbicides**

  - Corn and cotton plants engineered to produce a built-in insecticide are registered pesticides

  - Spraying of herbicide on herbicide-resistant crops resulted in a 527 million pound increase in herbicide use from 1996-2011

- **Grows huge amounts of single crops such as corn and soy repeatedly over large areas**

  - Sets the stage for food security issues, such as a lack of variety in food choices and increased vulnerability to pests or diseases that might spread through single crops

  - Predisposes us to health problems because single-crop foods produced in excessive amounts end up in unhealthy processed food products and factory-farmed meats

A GENETICALLY MODIFIED WORLD?

These basics about GMOs and the system of agriculture that goes with them are enough to convince many people to go non-GMO. But it gets still more troubling.

Genetic engineers want to completely change our world as we know it, creating a genetically modified existence in which nothing is as nature intended. About 140 of nature's living things are on the drawing board to become genetically modified. Here are just some of the new products biotechnology companies have developed and are pushing hard to get commercialized:

- **Genetically modified apple.** A Canadian firm, Okanagan Specialty Fruits, has developed a GM apple known as the Arctic Apple that is genetically engineered to prevent oxidation, or turning brown when sliced or bruised. The company is using a new genetic engineering technique known as "gene silencing." Scientists say that not only does the "Franken-apple" offer no real benefit to consumers, but also the technology used to create it is risky and inherently dangerous.[59] It is completely unknown what "gene silencing" could do if people or animals ate apples created with this new technique, and of course both conventional and organic apple orchards could become contaminated from this foreign GMO apple pollen.[60] Apples are the second most popular fruit in the United States, and there is stiff opposition to this product from both consumers and non-GMO apple growers.[61]

- **Genetically modified salmon.** AquaBounty Technologies, Inc., has genetically engineered salmon by inserting a fragment of DNA from an ocean pout fish (a type of eel), along with a growth hormone gene from Chinook Pacific salmon, into a fertilized Atlantic salmon egg. The result? Salmon that produce growth hormone year-round instead of only during warm weather. This form of genetic engineering is supposed to allow the fish to reach market weight in just 18 months, instead of the usual three years. According to evidence from a 2013 peer-reviewed study, genetically engineered salmon can breed with wild trout and create offspring that grow even faster and can overwhelm wild fish, greatly raising concerns about environmental damage.

Close to 2 million Americans wrote the FDA opposing the introduction of this so-called "Frankenfish." More than three-quarters of Americans don't want it, and 59 grocery retailers have committed to not selling GM salmon if it is approved.[62] Canadian environmental groups also don't want this GM fish: They have taken the Canadian federal government to court for permitting the manufacture of GM salmon in Canada.[63] If allowed on the market, GM salmon would be the first genetically engineered animal approved for human consumption and would likely open the gates to the approval of more GM fish and other GM animals.

- **Genetically modified mosquitos.** Oxitec, a biotechnology company from the United Kingdom, has developed genetically engineered mosquitos in an attempt to reduce mosquito populations and limit the spread of disease such as dengue fever. The company wants to release its GM mosquitos in Key West, Florida, but there has been strong opposition from the public.[64] The GM mosquitos are bred in a lab by injecting mosquito eggs with a killer gene. Only GM male mosquitos are intentionally released into the wild to breed with non-GM females to produce offspring genetically programmed to die well before reproductive age. But as critics point out, and Oxitec acknowledges, the release of a small number of GM females, which are the ones that bite and spread disease, cannot be avoided.

- **Genetically modified trees.** GM trees have already started with GM papayas and the GM apple described above. But biotech companies want to go much further down the path of the flawed industrial agriculture system. They want to replace natural trees in forests with trees genetically engineered to have herbicide tolerance, insecticide production, and other traits to accelerate proliferation of large-scale, industrial tree plantations and increase profits for a handful of corporations—biotechnology companies and paper, biofuel, lumber, and energy businesses.

Trees are more complex organisms than agricultural crops and have much longer lives. Additionally, GM trees are much more likely to cross-pollinate with wild varieties, which means untested GM genes might not be contained and could move into our national parks and forests, changing their character and landscape forever. According to the Sierra Club's website, "The possibility that the new genes spliced into [GM] trees will interfere with natural forests isn't a hypothetical risk but a certainty."[65] In the documentary *A Silent Forest*, Anne Petermann, co-director of the Global Justice Ecology Project, explains it this way: "[GM] trees are truly the greatest threat to the world's remaining native forests since the invention of the chainsaw."[66]

The USDA is currently considering whether to allow the unrestricted planting of ArborGen's GMO eucalyptus trees. According to the Center for Food Safety, these trees pose a number of dangers, including the strong likelihood for contamination of non-GM trees, massive consumption of water, high flammability, and unknown impacts on wildlife species.[67]

THE PRO-INDUSTRY STANCE OF THE U.S.

There's one more important piece of information to know and it may rock your world like it did mine: The United States has a pro-GMO agenda, and U.S. government agencies in charge of protecting our environment, our agriculture system, and our foods—the Environmental Protection Agency (EPA), the Department of Agriculture (USDA), and the Food and Drug Administration (FDA)—not only repeatedly favor industry over the people's will but actively promote GM technology.

For example, the USDA gave AquaBounty, the GM salmon company, a $500,000 research grant in 2011 and gave Recombinetics, Inc, $500,000 to develop a genetically modified pig.[68] [69] It also heavily subsidizes large agrichemical corporations that produce genetically modified crops such as corn and soy. In many cases, former employees of biotech companies now hold key positions at the EPA, USDA, and FDA overseeing key decisions about genetically modified foods. Michael Taylor, who earlier in his career worked as a lawyer for King and Spalding, a law firm that represented GM seed giant Monsanto, was the FDA's Deputy Commissioner of Policy when the official FDA policy on GMOs was developed.[70] Later, Taylor became the Vice President for Public Policy of Monsanto, and he currently is back at the FDA as the Deputy Commissioner for Foods and Veterinary Medicine.[71] (Many who learn this call the situation "the fox guarding the hen house.")

GOING AGAINST THE GRAIN
OF OUR CURRENT FOOD SYSTEM

Perhaps by now, you realize why there's a non-GMO movement growing like wildfire. When people really understand the full picture involving the agricultural system behind producing GM foods and the persistent hijacking of our natural foods, they begin to see how problematic GMOs are in the long run for our food security and for the planet.

As pesticide policy expert Charles Benbrook, Ph.D., said in *The Future of Food* documentary, meaningful change in our food system will only happen when the American public and farmers stand up and say:

> Wait a minute. We just don't want to go any further down this road. ... We're a government of the people, for the people, and by the people, and "Hey, we're the people. We don't want to go there."

The more people learn about GM foods, the more they realize that avoiding GM foods is a key step in a movement to wrestle control of our food away from chemical corporations that have a different vision of the world than that of virtually all of us everyday citizens. When people understand the situation, they realize that we the people must take control of our food supply system away from junk food, chemical, and agribusiness corporations that care only about maximizing profit, not about the public good. As Zack Kaldveer, former Assistant Media Director for the Organic Consumers Association, said in a 2014 online GMO education conference:

> As a country and as a planet, we're going to have to make a choice: continue pursuing a catastrophic genetically modified food future, or begin the rapid transition to a sustainable organic one.

When we go against the chemical-intensive system that was pushed on us without most of our knowledge and choose to purchase healthy, non-GMO, organic foods as much as we possibly can, we cast our vote against a genetically modified food future and for a sustainable food future. That's exactly what growing numbers of people are doing.

But there's still other important information to know. In the next chapter, you'll learn about the health risks of GMOs, which further explain why so many are opting out of eating GM foods.

Chapter 3:

Risky Business: The Health Risks
of Genetically Modified Foods

Almost all of us have been eating genetically modified foods without realizing it. What we didn't know we've been eating may be harming our health, as you'll soon read.

You won't hear the information in this chapter from the government or from corporations that produce GM foods, just like they kept it from us that GM ingredients were secretly added into our food supply decades ago.

When trying to evaluate the health effects of GM foods, it's important to understand that virtually no research has been done on humans. Most animal research that has been done is performed by the biotech industry or affiliated scientists and is based on short-term studies. Furthermore, independent scientists who go public with research that raises concern about GMOs are penalized by having their funding taken away, losing their jobs, or being publicly attacked, discredited, threatened, or denied tenure.[72] [73]

Evidence that we know isn't influenced by the biotech industry comes from animal research from independent scientists not affiliated with the industry, case studies of patients (like my client Marcia whose story I covered in the Introduction), and personal experiences of farmers, ranchers and veterinarians who have seen amazing health improvements in animals when their feed is switched from GMO to non-GMO.

WHAT ANIMAL RESEARCH SHOWS

In 2009, after studying animal research on GM foods, the American Academy of Environmental Medicine (AAEM), an international organization of physicians, said that there are serious health risks associated with eating GM foods. Those risks include:

- Infertility

- Immune system problems

- Accelerated aging

- Disruption of insulin and cholesterol regulation

- Gastrointestinal problems

- Changes in the liver, spleen, and gastrointestinal tract

"There is more than a casual association between GM foods and adverse health effects. There is causation," as defined by recognized scientific criteria, the academy concluded.

The AAEM became so concerned by its findings that the group called for a moratorium on GM foods and urged doctors to prescribe non-GMO diets for all patients. The AAEM said that doctors are probably seeing negative health effects in their patients right now from GM foods but not realizing that GM foods are major contributors to various health conditions.[74] [75]

WARNINGS FROM DOCTORS

In 2009, after evaluating the animal research, the AAEM, an international organization of physicians, said genetically modified foods posed serious health risks. The organization called for a moratorium on GM foods and urged physicians to advise patients to avoid GM foods.

The academy concluded: "There is more than a casual association between GM foods and adverse health effects. There is causation."

RESULTS FROM LONG-TERM ANIMAL STUDIES

Results of the first animal trial examining the long-term effects of exposure to Roundup-tolerant GM corn and the complete herbicide formulation Roundup were published in the scientific journal *Food and Chemical Toxicology* in 2012. The study lasted two years, the average lifespan of the rats used in the study. The rats were fed GM corn and received amounts of Roundup that reflected the normal amount we would receive from eating a typical diet. The type of corn used was NK603, a Monsanto-patented variety of GM corn that's grown across North America and widely fed to animals and humans.

The study linked varying levels of both Roundup and the NK603 corn to mammary tumors in female rats and severe liver and kidney damage in male rats. As a result of the massive breast tumors and liver and kidney damage in the rats fed NK603 corn, up to 50 percent of the male rats and 70 percent of the female rats died prematurely, compared with only 30 percent and 20 percent in the control group.[76]

Word about this study and photos of the disfiguring tumors in the rats spread quickly through social media, prompting many people to go non-GMO for good. But about a year later, the publishers of that journal did something unprecedented: They retracted the study, even though they admitted that the study authors had committed no mistakes or deliberate deception—criteria typically needed to publish a retraction. The publishers said they had concerns about the number of rats and type of rat used in the study.

However, as Professor Gilles-Eric Séralini, the lead researcher, and his supporters pointed out, the offending strain of rat (the Sprague-Dawley) is used routinely in the United States, sometimes by Monsanto itself, to study the carcinogenicity and chronic toxicity of chemicals. It also is the same type of rat that was used in a 2004 study by Monsanto finding the same strain of GMO corn (NK603) safe after measuring its effects in the same number of rats for three months only. So, Séralini's study used the same type and number of rats and the same type of corn as Monsanto did in one of its studies, just for a longer period of time—the average lifespan of that type of rat.

More than a hundred scientists protested the journal's retraction, writing:

> This arbitrary, groundless retraction of a published, thoroughly peer-reviewed paper is without precedent in the history of scientific publishing, and raises grave concerns over the integrity and impartiality of science.

SUMMARY OF RECENT LONG-TERM ANIMAL STUDIES

- **A 2012 study involving rats given GM corn and Roundup for their lifetimes**

  - Varying degrees of GM corn and Roundup were linked to liver and kidney damage in male rats and breast tumors in female rats

  - Premature death in 50% of male rats (vs. 30% in the control group)

  - Premature death in 70% of female rats (vs. 20% in the control group)

  - A year after being published, the study was controversially retracted. It was republished in *Environmental Sciences Europe* a year later.

- **A 2013 study involving pigs fed GM or non-GM corn and soy feed for their lifetimes**

  - Higher rate of severe stomach inflammation in those fed GM feed

  - Uteri of the female pigs fed GMOs were much larger.

The scientists said their concerns were heightened in part by the appointment of ex-Monsanto employee Richard E. Goodman to the newly created post of Biotechnology Paper Editor at the journal. They also said they will no longer publish, purchase, or review articles in Elsevier publications like *Food and Chemical Toxicology* unless the retraction is reversed.[77]

Both the French Food Safety Agency and the European Food Safety Authority agree with Séralini that additional long-term safety assessment should be done on GM foods: On June 28, 2013, the European Commission announced it was spending 3 million Euros to fund a two-year carcinogenicity study on the same NK603 variety of corn used in the Séralini study. Furthermore, in June 2014, Séralini and his research team announced they republished the study in the open-sourced, peer-reviewed journal *Environmental Sciences Europe*. Now anyone can view the results.[78]

(Keep in mind that Séralini is not the first researcher whose work has been criticized or called into question after finding results that raise serious concern about GM foods. Other scientists who have found disturbing research results and faced similar attempts at disaccreditation include Arpad Pusztai, Ignacio Chapela, Irina Ermakova, and Andres Carrasco.[79])

In 2013, results from another long-term study on GMOs were published. The study found that pigs fed a mixed GM corn and GM soy diet had a higher rate of severe stomach inflammation than pigs fed a non-GMO corn and soy diet. Uteri of the female pigs fed GMOs also were much larger. The effects on pigs eating GMOs were evaluated because pigs have a similar gastrointestinal tract to humans.[80] Disturbing results seen in animal studies are key reasons why many people, including some former pro-GMO advocates, have now become anti-GMO advocates.

FROM PRO-GMO TO ANTI-GMO

Thierry Vrain, Ph.D., is a retired soil biologist and genetic engineer who had worked for Agriculture Canada, the Canadian equivalent of our Department of Agriculture, for 30 years. Part of his job involved being a spokesperson assuring the public that genetically engineered crops and foods were safe. "I breathed genetic engineering all day long and could not understand why people were concerned," he says.

Since retiring close to a dozen years ago and learning about scientific evidence ignored by most biotech industry promoters and government regulators, Vrain has reversed his position and now warns of the dangers from GMOs. The following are major concerns that led him to change his mind:

- **Animals fed GM foods get ill.** Health problems in animals have been found in numerous independent studies, including the research of Arpad Pusztai, Ph.D., a top toxicologist who was commissioned by the European Union (EU) to design a protocol to test GM crops for the EU. In Pusztai's 1998 research, rats fed GM potatoes engineered to produce their own insecticide developed immune system damage, enlarged pancreases and intestines, partial atrophy of the liver, and increased cell growth in the stomach lining and small and large intestine within less than four months. The results were so alarming that Pusztai went public with his findings to caution both the European administrations and the public about GM foods. Pusztai was fired from his job, but word about his warnings spread, prompting such widespread public protest that major food companies pulled GM ingredients from their European food products. Pusztai's research was later thoroughly reviewed by peers and published in one of the most prestigious medical research journals, The Lancet.[81]

- **New proteins, often called rogue proteins, are formed in GM foods.** When Vrain worked for the Canadian government, he was not aware that inserting a new gene could lead to the formation of proteins that are different from the proteins expected by genetic engineers. But the Human Genome Project found that any gene can code for more than one protein, and inserting a gene anywhere in a plant eventually creates rogue proteins. Some of these proteins can be allergenic or toxic.

- **The herbicide that goes hand in hand with GM foods is a cause for "alarm," says Vrain.** Almost all GM crops are engineered to resist the herbicide Roundup, and this is by far the factor that causes the former genetic engineer the most concern. The herbicide that is used now in astoundingly higher amounts is a chelator: It grabs and binds many metal ions (electrically charged atomic particles) and therefore interferes with numerous enzyme proteins, which contain metal atoms and are needed to carry on life processes in living things. In other words, glyphosate, the active ingredient in Roundup, insidiously impairs life, according to Vrain.

  The herbicide also kills bacteria, including good bacteria, in healthy soil. Both of these effects can create a desertification process, causing healthy soil to become unhealthy. After a few years of using the technology, farmers notice that their soil becomes less and less "alive," Vrain explains. Additionally, Roundup is a hormone disruptor and has been implicated in the development of several diseases. The herbicide is dangerous, and it's badly contaminating our agriculture in ways that could cause a severe health epidemic, says Vrain.

- **Antibiotic-resistance genes in GM foods are spreading into soil and water.** In most GM foods currently on the market, antibiotic-resistance genes typically have been inserted as markers to determine in which cells the bacterial genes have taken hold. This means that every cell of that engineered plant contains an antibiotic-resistance gene. Based on this technology, Vrain estimates that there are an astounding number—10 to the power of 19—of antibiotic-resistance genes out in our environment today. Antibiotic-resistance genes are not only in GM foods we eat, but are picked up by bacteria in the soil through lateral or horizontal gene transfer; then they make their way into water in the soil, and possibly into the local ditches, streams, and rivers, according to Vrain. Exposure to so many antibiotic- resistance genes should be a big worry for everyone because it might exacerbate the growing epidemic of antibiotic-resistant germs and reduce options for controlling infections.

- **GMOs don't help us with our agriculture problems.** "We hear that GMOs are necessary for reducing pesticides, for increasing yields, for feeding the world, for lowering the cost of food. These statements are not based in science. They're not based in reality at all. There are many global agencies, including the United Nations and the Food and Agriculture Organization of the United Nations, which have come out saying exactly the opposite, that this is not the technology of the future and will not feed the world," says Vrain.

He believes that genetically engineered food should have never been allowed on our grocery shelves and that the genetic engineering of our food has gone so far in the United States and Canada that labeling GM foods is not enough to protect us from the problems posed by GMOs in the food system. Vrain now favors a GMO ban in agriculture and a grassroots revolution to change our current GMO-based food system.

Health Improvements on Non-GMO Foods

Our piecing together the picture of what GMOs might be doing to our health goes far beyond what has been shown in animal studies and the numerous health issues that concern Vrain. As a result of the AAEM recommendations, new studies that have been published in recent years, and consistent, tireless education from non-GMO advocates, particularly Institute for Responsible Technology Executive Director Jeffrey M. Smith, thousands of practitioners are now prescribing non-GMO diets—in other words, a return to *real* food—for their patients and clients. Individuals are increasingly coming forward with stories of dramatic health improvements, including lessening and/or clearing up of digestive issues, skin conditions, migraines, weight problems, fatigue and more, from switching to a non-GMO diet.

Many who avoid GMOs do so by switching to organic food. Some also eliminate processed foods and specific food categories at the same time. Because so many factors are involved, it's difficult to know whether it's a non-GMO diet or another healthy dietary change that is responsible for the health improvements people experience.

But additional evidence from veterinarians and farmers who made only one change—switching from GMO to non-GMO feed for their animals—more definitively points to eating GMOs leading to health problems and not eating them clearing up health issues. In a November 2013 Institute for Responsible Technology blog post below, Smith described this evidence:[82]

> [In pigs and cows taken off GMO feed,]... Death rates dropped, stillborn rates were down, litter size was up, and overall health improved. One farmer was ecstatic about the huge increase in milk production in his herd; another described how healthy his pigs looked—even down to reduced blood shot eyes.

The vets I spoke with had all been in practice long before 1996, when GMOs were introduced. Each had his stories about the surge in diseases and disorders after GM feed came on the scene. One told me that the jump in dog and cat allergies correlated exactly with the introduction of GM pet food. Whenever he switched his allergic animals to an organic (non-GMO) brand, their symptoms such as itching would usually disappear. Others described inflammation, infections, and gastrointestinal disorders.

Both vets and farmers saw differences *inside* GM-fed animals during autopsies or butchering, including liver damage, stomach ulcers, discoloration, and an awful stench. One farmer said that after seeing the alterations inside GM-fed animals, he and his wife started a strict non-GMO policy for their family's meat.

In other words, veterinarians and farmers see animals get better on non-GMO diets, and the animals tend to improve from the same types of diseases and disorders that lab animals developed from eating GMOs—gastrointestinal problems, immune system problems, reproductive problems, and organ trouble.

Pet owners also are noticing similar health improvements when they switch their pets to non-GMO feed. Two women from Prescott, Arizona, describe their experiences with pets below.

Two Testimonials From Pet Owners

A year ago I helped care for two Teacup Chihuahuas ages 8 and 2 years and had been feeding them a commercial corn-based dog food. I decided to do an experiment and bought some organic dog food called Organix from a company named Castor & Pollux. I put both of the foods in front of them and both dogs chose the organic food. I switched to feeding them the organic dog food regularly, and the dogs experienced more energy, became more playful, and had much better digestion and elimination than they ever did before. I am sold. I am convinced that eliminating GMOs from the dogs' diets upgraded their quality of life. Yes, the organic food costs more. However, the benefits over time far outweigh the initial investment.

– Celia

About a month and a half ago I put my dog and myself on an organic non-GMO diet. He had suffered from allergies, which caused problems on his skin and paws and in his ears for ten years starting every spring. I was determined to get rid of the allergies and spent a couple of days researching dog foods. Around this time I was fortunate to watch a movie on GMOs and the big elephant in the room became apparent.

After putting him on certified organic dog food (which of course was non-GMO), I was pretty shocked to see that within two days of his new diet, his immune system began to heal, his allergies went away, and all the licking, chewing, biting, and scratching had/has stopped! I also experienced a lot of healing of various problems in myself that were mostly the result of chemotherapy eight years ago. These included bowel problems, allergies, depression, low energy level, and aches and pains. If I don't eat non-GMO, those problems return.

After much research and anecdotal evidence regarding animals, it's apparent to me that using only non-GMO foods is obvious for survival and health. I find it upsetting that this corruption and manipulation of our food supply was ever allowed in the first place and I feel that this is a "cancer" that is slowly spreading across the globe and must be stopped.

– Ginny

THE OUTDATED HYPOTHESIS
BEHIND GENETIC ENGINEERING

In genetic engineering, a gene is inserted into the DNA of a plant, with the goal of making a protein that creates a specific new trait in the plant. Genetic engineering is based on the "one gene-one protein hypothesis" from the 1940s that each gene is coded for, or gives order to the cell to create, a single protein.

The Human Genome Project completed in 2002 showed that this hypothesis is wrong, according to former pro-GMO scientist Thierry Vrain, Ph.D.[83] It's now known that that the vast majority of genes do not code for just one protein. Genes collaborate to make proteins and can make more than one protein depending on the environment in the cell.[84] Some genes make many proteins, which are not only the building blocks of all the tissues and organs in our bodies, but also form countless substances vital for proper body functioning, from antibodies that fight infections to hormones that regulate everything from metabolism to fertility.

When foreign genes are inserted, the functioning of genes may be altered, creating damaged, mutated, new, or unknown proteins, which may be allergenic, toxic, or antinutritional.

UNINTENDED CONSEQUENCES THAT POSE HEALTH RISKS

How might GMOs contribute to so many different health problems suggested by the animal research, and why do animals and people get better eating non-GMO food? There hasn't been enough independent research to fully answer these questions. But we do know a few things about the nature of genetic engineering itself and the two main types of genetically modified crops.

The very process of genetically engineering plants—inserting foreign genes into the DNA of the plant—is inexact and causes unintended consequences that pose health risks. "The general public has the false impression that genetic engineering is precise. In truth, it's sub-microscopic shooting from the hip, resulting in unpredictable, and potentially dangerous changes in the organisms' DNA and the health properties of food," says Robin Bernhoft, M.D., former president of the American Academy of Environmental Medicine, in an Institute for Responsible Technology informational brochure.[85]

Jeffrey Smith, who is also the author and movie producer of *Genetic Roulette*, describes it this way: "Irrespective of what particular gene you insert, the very process of creating a GMO results in massive collateral damage in the plant, which can increase toxins, allergens, carcinogens, and antinutrients." Remember that the FDA's own scientists warned that GM foods could lead to unexpected side effects, including allergens, toxins, new diseases, and nutritional problems, and urged their superiors to require long-term safety studies on GM foods. But no one acted on the scientists' warnings.

OTHER WAYS THE MAIN TYPES OF GMOS MAY DISRUPT HEALTH

Insecticide-producing genetically modified crops (primarily a type of corn called Bt corn) contains a toxin called Bt toxin that breaks open pores and creates small holes in the cells of insects' digestive tracts, leading to the death of insects such as the European corn borer. Genetic engineers claim that Bt toxin is quickly destroyed in our stomach, and even if it survived, it wouldn't cause reactions in humans or mammals. But new research shows Bt toxin from GM corn creates similar holes in human cells.[86] Researchers and in-the-know practitioners theorize that it may do similar damage in our gastrointestinal tracts, contributing to a wide range of digestive problems that have been on the rise, and promoting permeable intestines, commonly called "leaky gut." This condition can lead to an immune system attack on undigested proteins, inflammatory reactions and other symptoms of a hypersensitized immune system, as well as autoimmune reactions such as celiac disease.[87]

We also have to consider the effects of herbicide, specifically glyphosate, the active ingredient in the world's bestselling weed killer Roundup. About 85 percent of all genetically engineered plants worldwide are herbicide tolerant—designed to tolerate high levels of herbicides, glyphosate-based Roundup in particular—and as I explained in Chapter 2, herbicide has been used in astoundingly higher amounts since the introduction of herbicide-resistant genetically modified crops, meaning more herbicide residues are on (and absorbed into) the herbicide-resistant foods we eat.

The biotech industry claims that glyphosate is safe for humans. But research suggests otherwise. Reports from areas of South America where GM Roundup Ready soy is grown and sprayed with high doses of herbicide link Roundup or glyphosate exposure to increases in birth defects and some cancers.[88] A 2010 study found that glyphosate causes malformations in frog and chicken embryos at doses far lower than those used in agricultural spraying.[89] Other studies have pointed to Roundup disrupting endocrine (or hormone) function.[90]

Don Huber, Ph.D., Professor Emeritus of Soil Pathology at Purdue University, who has 50 years of experience in plant physiology and microbiology, has put himself on the line in recent years by exposing a few key ways he believes glyphosate is harmful.[91] [92] [93] First and foremost, glyphosate was originally developed as a chelating agent. In other words, it grabs elements such as vital nutrients and makes them unavailable, depriving plants of essential minerals needed for healthy functioning, weakening the plants' defenses, and promoting the diseases in the soil that end up killing the plant, according to Huber.

Tissue tests have documented deficiencies in manganese, copper, and zinc in glyphosate-treated plants. When animals eat those nutrient-deficient plants, the animals become nutrient deficient, weak and sick, and when we eat animals and plants that are nutrient deficient, we may become nutrient deficient, weak, and sick. "Those deficiencies are very well documented as being factors in animal diseases as well as in human diseases," Huber explained in the movie *Genetic Roulette*.

Glyphosate is also an effective bactericide or antibiotic: It kills vitally important beneficial soil bacteria, cow gut bacteria, and human gut bacteria, setting up bacterial imbalances that disrupt health, according to Huber.[94] [95] Intestinal microflora imbalances—or imbalances of the good and bad bacteria in our gut—are known to be involved in many different health conditions, including gluten intolerance, obesity, and the cluster of insulin-resistance-related heart disease risk factors known as metabolic syndrome that I wrote about in *Syndrome X*.[96] [97]

I've seen a decline in children's health, and children are not as healthy as their parents.

Genetically engineered foods contain new proteins that children have not been previously exposed to. I believe this may be responsible in part for the profound increase in allergies and immune dysfunction that I am witnessing.

– Michelle Perro, M.D., integrative pediatrician, Institute for Health & Healing in San Francisco and Greenbrae, CA

From a nutritionist's point of view, this little-known information about glyphosate is startling. Any factor that may contribute to the development of leaky gut and promote imbalances of good and bad bacteria in the gut can set people up for a multitude of health problems. These two factors alone could play a big part in recent increases in many conditions, including gluten sensitivity, allergies, asthma, and autism. Consider the story of Nora who had been a very sick little child.

NORA'S STORY

When she was only 2 months old, Nora started to have what her mother Lisa describes as "goopy and crusty," chronic severe nasal congestion and "not normal" baby poop that ranged from being runny and watery to looking like green mucus. Nora was sick in many ways. She didn't look well and her face was puffy. Even though she was exclusively breast fed, Nora experienced adverse symptoms—reactions to foods such as soy and milk products that her mother Lisa ate—so Lisa removed those foods from her diet to help Nora feel better.

But Nora's extremely concerning health issues continued. Right after she began eating solid foods, Nora developed one terrible ear infection after another and was put on antibiotics nine different times between January and June of 2013. On the advice of a top ear, nose, and throat pediatrician in their area, Nora's parents decided to have their daughter's adenoids removed. However, a few months later Nora was sick again and couldn't get better. Several months later, when the family was traveling a lot, Nora was so sick, sometimes screaming at night from the pain of yet another ear infection, that she had to be taken for urgent and emergency room care twice in two weeks.

It was at that point that Lisa took her toddler to see Michelle Perro, M.D. The experienced pediatrician suggested removing GMOs, pesticides, and other toxins from Nora's food by putting the young girl on an organic diet. Lisa felt overwhelmed by that suggestion and her husband was skeptical and didn't like the idea of spending more money on organic foods. But because Nora was so sick, both parents decided they had to try it.

The first major change they made was switching Nora's favorite cereal to an organic, non-GMO version. Within 48 hours of making that change, something amazing happened: Nora's longstanding congestion cleared up. All of a sudden, other symptoms dramatically improved: Nora started using more words; the puffiness in her face went away; her eyes became brighter; she started sleeping through the night again; and she became much happier and more fun to be around. She hasn't had another ear infection since her diet was changed.

"It was just unbelievable the difference the change in diet made because she had been sick for so long," says Lisa. "Nora went from being so sick that we were having multiple emergency medical visits to being like a new little girl now. I can't overstate the difference in how dramatic the change in her was."

"We're convinced that going non-GMO and organic made all the difference for Nora," adds Lisa, who has become so convinced that the whole family is now avoiding GMOs and going organic as much as possible.

THE GMO CONNECTION TO FOOD ALLERGIES

There is clearly evidence that implicates eating GMOs in many different health conditions. But as a nutritionist who advises many clients with food allergies, I think it's important to share specific evidence pointing to a GMO connection to food allergies. You'll recall that the FDA's own scientists warned that genetically modified foods could lead to new allergens. Also, animal research found that mice fed Bt toxin (which is what insecticide-producing corn makes) reacted directly and also became sensitive to formerly harmless compounds.[98] [99]

As I explained in *Going Against the Grain*, a study published in *The New England Journal of Medicine* in 1996 found that inserting a foreign gene into the DNA of a plant can turn a nonallergenic food into an allergy-producing food. Researchers at the University of Nebraska, Lincoln, discovered that people with a sensitivity to Brazil nuts (who didn't have a sensitivity to soybeans) became allergic to genetically engineered soybeans.[100] Fortunately, based on those findings, the company discontinued the development of the GM soybean, but "the next case could be less ideal, and the public less fortunate," according to a companion editorial in the same issue of *The New England Journal of Medicine*.[101]

Also consider what we know about soy. Before it began to be genetically modified, soy was already a top food allergen, but the incidence of soy allergies dramatically increased in the United Kingdom after it began to be genetically modified.[102] [103] There could be several reasons for that, with one of the key ones being that cooked GM soy contains higher amounts of an allergen. One study found that cooked GM soy contains seven times more trypsin inhibitor, a known soy allergen, than cooked non-GM soy.[104] [105]

The number of people who have food allergies is growing, but there is no clear answer why, according to Food Allergy Research & Education. Allergy specialists who are up to speed on the research I've described in this chapter are considering the correlation between the rise in allergies—and other conditions—and the introduction of genetically engineered foods.[106] According to a study released in 2013 by the Centers for Disease Control and Prevention, food allergies among children increased approximately 50 percent between 1997 and 2011.[107] Genetically modified crops were introduced into our food supply in 1996, right before this upward trend in childhood food allergies began.

CORN ALLERGIES

As I described in the Introduction, I first learned about GMO contamination of foods and allergies to GM foods in 2000 and 2001 when I was compiling information for *Going Against the Grain.* A type of pesticide-producing corn called StarLink corn that concerned the EPA was approved for animal feed but was not approved for human consumption—but it ended up in our food anyway. A coalition of environmental groups, including Friends of the Earth and the Center for Food Safety, essentially did the work our government agencies should have been doing, tested foods, and discovered StarLink corn in store-bought taco shells in September 2000.[108]

When the StarLink contamination of commercial corn products was reported by the U.S. media, thousands of people complained to food companies about reactions they had, but the companies and the FDA didn't follow up on those complaints. Only 51 individuals filled out the paperwork necessary to register their reactions with the FDA, and their symptoms ranged from abdominal pain and diarrhea or skin rashes to a very small number having life-threatening reactions.[109] CBS News interviewed a woman who had a severe reaction that sent her to the hospital.

StarLink corn was withdrawn from the market but many types of insecticide-producing Bt corn have been introduced since then and are now in our food supply. Corn allergy used to be considered rare, but reactions to corn appear to be on the rise, according to a number of reports.[110] [111] [112] Several corn-allergy websites have been created on the Internet in recent years. An allergy to corn has become so much more common than it used to be that author Kim Koeller included advice for dealing with corn allergy, in addition to the eight other common allergies, in the recent edition of her book *Let's Eat Out Around the World: Gluten Free and Allergy Free.*

Allergies to corn were even addressed in the August 2013 issue of *Elle* magazine, which has a circulation of more than 1 million readers. The author of the article, Caitlin Shetterly, describes how she had pain radiating throughout her body, rashes, exhaustion, constant head cold symptoms, and diarrhea, and she saw numerous doctors and tried many therapies.

She eventually visited an allergist named Paris Mansmann, M.D., who told her he believes that changes in the DNA of corn act as allergenic proteins that provoke the overproduction of eosinophils, a pro-inflammatory type of white blood cell that leads to inflammatory conditions throughout the body, many symptoms, and a multi-systemic disorder. Her doctor recommended that she remove all corn from her diet, and when she did, most of her symptoms went away, some fairly quickly.[113]

The experience described by Shetterly closely resembles that of my client Marcia, whose story I shared in the Introduction. Although Marcia had been eating gluten free for eight years, she continued to experience health problems across the board, and she consistently had a high eosinophil count. I recommended that she try taking all direct sources of GMOs out of her diet. She did, and she recovered her health. (Make sure to refer back to the Introduction to learn about the many dramatic ways Marcia's health improved.)

When Marcia and I read the *Elle* article and compared her experience with the information about how an allergy to GM corn may produce wide-ranging symptoms, we suspected that's exactly what Marcia had—and why avoiding GMOs, and perhaps hidden GM corn in particular, was a key answer to recovering her health.

CHOOSING REAL FOODS
OVER INDUSTRY-MANIPULATED FOODS

Throughout this chapter, I have described the most important GMO-related health evidence so far that I have seen as a nutritionist. Though there aren't a lot of long-term independent studies on the effects of GMOs, I'm sure you can see there is more than enough evidence from various sources to exercise caution.

When it comes to health, it's always better to be safe than sorry. Remember: Eating non-GMO is not a radical diet. It's simply eating time-tested real food. There's nothing controversial or unscientific about that.

Based on what I have seen in my practice, coupled with a reported increase in cases, corn allergies appear to be a special risk that more people are starting to identify. Wide-ranging symptoms and a high eosinophil count may be red flags that your body is allergically reacting to GM corn and perhaps to other GM foods.

It's important to understand that disease builds over time from eating the wrong foods. History is full of examples of newfangled "foods" being added to the mass food supply—industrially produced pseudo-foods such as white sugar, white flour, vegetable oils, and partially hydrogenated oils—that people accept and eat, and then their health slowly deteriorates.

Take partially hydrogenated oil loaded with trans-fats. Crisco vegetable shortening, which is made of partially hydrogenated oil, was first sold in grocery stores in 1911. Margarines and processed carbohydrate snack foods containing those same trans-fats followed, and over time, eating products with those industry-tinkered fats was contributing to disease. A little less than 20 years ago, research showed that eating a lot of trans-fats found in partially hydrogenated oils doubled the risk of heart disease, yet those products still remained in our food supply. More than a decade ago, many consumers became savvy about the research on trans-fats and started to avoid them in the foods they bought. Yet, even today, the Centers for Disease Control and Prevention estimates that a further reduction of trans-fats in the food supply could prevent an additional 7,000 deaths from heart disease and up to 20,000 heart attacks each year.[114] Just imagine what would have happened if people had not eaten trans-fats from the beginning. An ounce of prevention is worth a pound of cure.

Take refined sugar. As with other GM crops like corn and soy, sugar production is subsidized, so it is added ubiquitously into many foods. But we now know that sugar overconsumption is an independent risk factor in cardiovascular disease, which includes heart attacks, strokes, and artery disease, as well as in type 2 diabetes, liver cirrhosis, and dementia—diseases all linked to metabolic syndrome, which involves unhealthy blood fat levels, hypertension, and insulin resistance.[115] It's difficult to avoid sugar because research points to it being addictive, but it's increasingly well known that avoiding sugar is vital for protecting ourselves from degenerative diseases.

It's time that we connect the dots and see the big picture that industry-tinkered food products are created for the benefit of the companies that make them, not for the benefit of our health. Industry-manipulated pseudo-foods are not the fuel we were designed to live on. It isn't surprising that those fake food products don't support and promote our health like God- or nature-given foods do.

We're about two decades into GMOs being added into our food supply without our knowledge. It's more important than ever that we avoid GMOs and get back to eating *real* food. One key reason is to support our health over the long term. But the situation we're in now is unlike any other. GMOs are different from all other industry-driven foods because they are life forms that spread in an open environment and invade and take over *real* foods, changing them forever.

If we want to protect the integrity of real foods to support good health for future generations, we have to consistently choose non-GMO *real* foods. If we take a stand now to prevent any more GMOs from entering our food supply, we will put a halt to going any further down a road to a genetically modified future for all of us. The stakes are high, which is why so many are so passionate about saying no to GMOs.

Chapter 4:

The Top 10 Reasons to Avoid GMOs

In the last two chapters, I pieced together basic information about GMOs and the risks they pose to our health, the environment, farmers, our food security, and the control of our food, presenting an overwhelming amount of information that GMOs are not in our best interest.

If it was a lot for you to grasp, I understand. The many issues associated with GMOs are complicated. The weight of the information is difficult to absorb and takes a long time for most people to process.

This chapter will keep things simple, quickly summarizing the main reasons so many people are shopping and eating non-GMO and organic. Here are the top ten reasons behind the growing trend to avoid GMO foods:

1) *The desire for pure food and to not be a "lab rat."* Many say they simply want to eat real food as nature intended, not "Frankenfoods," in which engineers artificially insert genes from completely different life forms into the DNA of food crops or animals to make genetically modified organisms that aren't tested and would never occur in nature.

2) *The desire to protect health.* Animal research indicates serious health risks from eating GM foods, including infertility, immune system problems, accelerated aging, dysfunction of regulation of cholesterol and insulin, organ damage, and tumors.[116] [117] [118] Some veterinarians and farmers have reported dramatic improvements in pet and livestock health, especially in reproductive and gastrointestinal issues, when animals are switched from GMO feed to non-GMO feed. Numerous people, too, are now reporting similar health improvements when they go non-GMO.[119]

3) ***The desire to favor nature over industry.*** Man can't outsmart Mother Nature. That's true when it comes to genetically modifying foods, refining sugar, flour, or oils, or developing partially hydrogenated oils or artificial sweeteners such as aspartame. More people are understanding that every time the food industry has dramatically altered real food or created artificial substitutes, it has been for the benefit of company profits, not for our health. More consumers are deciding to avoid all industry-manipulated pseudo-foods, including GM foods, to prevent disease over the long term.

4) ***The desire to avoid pesticides.*** About 85 percent of all genetically modified foods that are grown are engineered for herbicide tolerance, which has led to increased herbicide spraying, an epidemic of herbicide-resistant "super weeds," and an astounding 527 million more pounds of herbicide used in the first 16 years of genetically modified crops being grown in the United States.[120] That of course means that higher amounts of toxic herbicide are polluting our soil, air, and water, and more herbicide residues are ending up on and in almost all genetically modified foods.

5) ***The desire to be good stewards of the Earth and protect the environment.*** Pollen and seeds from GM crops can easily spread through the air and contaminate organic and non-GMO crops. Once released into the wild, the new foreign genes can't be cleaned up or recalled and can easily move to bacteria in soil and pollute it. Many don't want to use their purchasing dollars to support a GMO-based system that leads to genetic pollution of our planet and unforeseen, potentially catastrophic consequences that might arise from that.

6) ***The desire to protect bees and other wildlife.*** Neonicotinoid insecticides used in higher amounts on GM corn seeds have been implicated in colony collapse disorder in bees—a cause of great concern for a number of shoppers because bees pollinate approximately one-third of the foods we eat.[121] [122]

The Roundup herbicide that goes with most GM crops currently on the market has been shown to be dangerous and even deadly to many living things. It kills milkweed, a primary food source for Monarch butterflies, and other vegetation that birds and mammals use for food. Research has shown that Roundup can do significant harm to fish after low concentration exposures, and it's highly toxic to amphibians at levels below EPA standards for drinking water and at concentrations they may be exposed to during overspraying.[123][124] One study by University of Pittsburgh researcher Rick Relyea found that Roundup killed 98 percent of all tadpoles within three weeks and 79 percent of all frogs within one day.[125] In addition, pesticide-producing Bt crops harm non-target insects, including beneficial bugs (such as ladybugs/ladybirds and lacewings) and microorganisms in the soil; they also may harm insect-eating bird populations.[126][127] Many people want to avoid pesticide-laden GM foods to help protect numerous living creatures at risk from the harmful effects of the pesticides that go hand in hand with GM food production.

7) *The desire to withdraw business from GM seed companies.* Large agrichemical corporations, such as Monsanto, the developer of DDT, Agent Orange, and Roundup herbicide, are the companies that are buying seeds, genetically modifying them, patenting them so farmers can't save and exchange those seeds as they have done throughout history, and then harassing and suing farmers who accidentally as a result of wind drift get the companies' patented GM crops growing in their fields.[128][129][130] Many shoppers feel strongly that they do not want to use their money to purchase products made by companies that use these types of business practices.

8) *The desire to support local and organic food growers and ethical food companies that make quality products.* By moving away from mass-produced GMO-based foods and toward

locally grown produce and high-quality organic or heirloom food products, we use our dollars wisely by rewarding food producers who are working in concert with the planet and are producing food that keeps us healthy.

9) *The desire to contribute to a collective consumer rejection of GMOs, forcing them out of our food supply.* We can and must do this right now. We don't have to wait for a policy change such as labeling. Simply follow the information on how to go against GMOs in the second section of this book. If enough people individually avoid GMOs creating profit losses for major food manufacturers, those companies will quickly abandon GM ingredients. That happened in Europe: Food purveyors stopped using GM ingredients in the products they sold following widespread public protest after a scientist went public with research results showing harm in animals fed GM feed. If we stop buying GMOs and are vocal about why we're no longer buying them, companies will stop making them. Many are realizing that the consumer is still king and we *can* kick GM foods out of our food supply.

10) *The desire to take back our food, health, and planet.* To stop going any further down the road of a genetically modified future, the first step that's needed is a huge increase in public awareness of GMOs and using our consumer power to say no to GM foods. Once we get past the shock, discouragement, frustration, and anger we feel after learning what has been done to our food system without our knowledge or consent, we have to understand that it's not enough to simply say we reject the current genetically modified, industrialized agricultural system.

It's important to put our focus on and actions toward what we want to build in its place—a health-promoting, sustainable food system that works in concert with nature. We can do that by taking these actions:

- Buy more organic foods

- Purchase more locally produced, pesticide-free and GMO-free foods directly from farmers

- Grow our own foods from non-GMO organic seeds in gardens or even window sills

- Plant historical or heirloom seeds, save them, and pass them along to others to protect our seeds from corporate takeover

- Financially support non-profit groups that are working toward these goals

- Network with others to collectively protest and change laws and rulings that favor industry instead of a healthy food system and healthy planet for all of us.

With the vision of an organic, locally centered food system firmly in our hearts and minds, we can create the change in our food system that we seek. As anthropologist Margaret Mead famously said: "Never doubt that a small group of thoughtful, committed citizens can change the world. Indeed, it is the only thing that ever has."

SECTION 2:

How to Go Against GMOs

Chapter 5:

Preparing for the Challenges Involved in Going Against GMOs

If you're like most people who learn what I covered in Chapters 2 through 4—that GM foods benefit chemical corporations and provide us with no benefits and only serious risks and dangers—you're probably raring to kick genetically modified foods out of your diet. The basic information about GMOs speaks for itself and is very motivating, which is why so many are going non-GMO in record numbers.

However, the real scoop has been kept from the public for so long that many people still aren't aware of the truth about GM foods. You have to go against the grain of society and against the foods most people are eating to avoid GMOs. Fortunately, there are some tricks of the trade I can give you after more than two decades of counseling clients to go against the standard American diet to get you prepped and mentally, emotionally, and spiritually ready to avoid GM foods.

KNOW THAT YOUR THINKING AND YOUR LIFE WILL CHANGE

Now that you know the breadth and seriousness of the GMO problem (especially in the United States and Canada!), your world has probably been rocked. When you begin to learn the top genetically modified foods to avoid—even the top five (corn, canola, cottonseed, soy and sugar from sugar beets)—and find out how many convenience foods have ingredients derived from these GM foods, it gets even more mindboggling. You begin to realize that *GMOs are everywhere, in all diets, in all grocery stores (including natural food supermarkets), in all restaurants (except the rare 100% organic restaurant), and even in many foods sold at farmers' markets.*

Never again will you think about food in exactly the same way. Instead of assuming any food you pick up is automatically *food* without thinking about it, you now know that a lot of what's out there isn't *real* food anymore and getting pure, unadulterated food is something you have to consciously fight for and work at finding. Understanding these basic concepts is likely jolting to the way you've perceived the world for a long time.

This means that no matter what type of diet we eat, we all go through the same heavy challenges trying to avoid GMOs. That at first seems quite discouraging. On the other hand, it means we're all in the same boat and we're all in this together. If we each do our part to spread the word to more people and avoid GM foods as best we can, we can conquer the GMO problem far more quickly than we realize. The incredibly fast-growing non-GMO movement that is influencing major food companies to already start making changes is evidence of that.

START SOMEWHERE AND DO WHAT YOU CAN

Though ideally I recommend that all of us get back to eating organic non-GMO real food like our grandparents did, I realize that most of us can't eat 100 percent GMO free, at least not right away. Going non-GMO is such a radical departure from how most Americans eat that it's difficult to change longstanding buying and eating habits and learn new ones. It's important to be patient with the process and allow yourself time to make those changes.

Each of us has different circumstances in our lives. Some of us have financial constraints and fewer options of where to find GMO-free foods. Others are time-pressed, juggling different jobs, traveling or eating out a lot for business, or being a caregiver to a loved one. Many different factors may prevent us from eating completely GMO free 100 percent of the time.

The important point to keep in mind is: Going non-GMO doesn't have to be all or nothing. *Simply start somewhere, at the place that feels most right for you and your situation, and gradually work on removing more GM foods from your diet.* If you don't think you can do much, **commit to eating one non-GMO or all organic meal a day.**

Another beginning strategy is to **avoid the Big Five—sugar, corn, soy, canola and cottonseed oil**—what I call the "pesticide plants." They make up virtually all of the genetically modified foods in processed convenience items. If each of us does what he or she can—say, one person eats non-GMO 30 percent of the time, another eats non-GMO 50 percent of the time, another eats non-GMO 75 percent of the time, and another eats non-GMO 90 to even 100 percent of the time—each of us will contribute to a tipping point of consumer rejection that will eventually kick GMOs out of the market for good.

BE PATIENT WITH THE PROCESS OF GOING NON-GMO

Trying to avoid GMOs sometimes feels like maneuvering through a minefield. GM foods are so ubiquitous in our society that there will be times when you either knowingly or unknowingly eat GM foods you didn't want to eat. During those times, don't lose heart, get discouraged, and give up. Simply pick yourself up, stay positive, and get back on the non-GMO bandwagon as quickly as you can, preferably at the next meal.

Know that dietary mistakes are a natural part of learning, and backslides are especially common when we're under stress. Try to learn from mistakes you might make—for example, not planning ahead and not having enough readily available non-GMO food to eat during a busy, time-pressured week.

Keep in mind that changing longstanding habits typically is an up-and-down process. It's most difficult in the beginning when you first start to avoid GM foods. I promise you that as with all other styles of eating, it gets easier to avoid GMOs the more you do it. Many people initially thought following a gluten-free or grain-free diet was "impossible," but it's clearly not. Look how many people are now routinely eating that way. To successfully go non-GMO, stay focused on your long-term goal, keep at it, and don't let momentary slip-ups deter you.

CONTINUALLY REMIND YOURSELF WHY YOU'RE AVOIDING GMOs

Perhaps the most important step for going against GMOs long term is to understand the many health, environmental, farmers' rights, and food security reasons to avoid GM foods. By reading this book, you're well on your way toward that goal. I suggest you re-read sections of the book often as a way to counter all the pro-GMO hype and propaganda in our culture (such as the familiar refrain that "GMOs will feed the world") with some solid scientific evidence and sound reasoning. With all the pro-GMO forces out there, it's easy to get confused at times, but the best offense against pro-GMO pressure is a good defense of knowledge.

I don't want to be a guinea pig in an experiment in which I did not give my consent.

I don't want to spend my hard-earned money on fake foods that are benefitting chemical companies and polluting the planet.

What you've read so far should provide the incentive you need to start eating against GMOs. To continue avoiding GMOs, keep fortifying yourself with the reasons that are the most important to you. Try writing down motivating passages from the book on Post-It notes and place them on your computer or desk—or put a reminder on your cell phone.

Or stick one of the notes just shown—or a different one that you create yourself—on your refrigerator.

Keep updating and refreshing your knowledge about the subject by visiting non-GMO websites, subscribing to newsletters that cover non-GMO news, following non-GMO group Facebook pages, and watching in-depth documentaries, such as *Genetic Roulette* and *The Future of Food*. The more knowledge you have firmly in your mind about GM foods, the more motivated you will be to steadfastly avoid them.

Do What's Right For You

Have the courage to eat non-GMO and preferably organic food, which you now know is best for you and our society over the long term. That means being a little different and politely but firmly asking for or requesting non-GMO and organic food. Doing that may be initially uncomfortable, but the more you do it, the easier it becomes. Although no one likes to rock the boat if not necessary, we need to be fairly radical—or at least strong-minded in our opposition to GM foods—because radical changes that are not beneficial for us have been done to our food without our consent!

Be prepared that when you don't follow the pack, your friends and acquaintances may put heavy-duty pressure on you to eat the GM food they're eating. Don't let this deter you. If you can't stomach what has been done to our food, there is no reason why you should have to eat chemical-laden GM food simply because that's what your friends are eating.

Keep in mind that sharing positive experiences with people you love is more important than eating the same food. Don't push too hard against others who aren't on your same wavelength on the GMO issue, and have a good attitude about avoiding the foods most others are eating. You just may get people curious and wanting to know more about GMOs.

To paraphrase something Robyn O'Brien, author of *The Unhealthy Truth*, says, taking a stand against GMOs (and other newfangled, toxic ingredients in our food supply) is the most patriotic thing you can do to get our food and country back on the right track. Some of your friends and family members may not at first understand why you're taking such a strong stand against what seems like everyday food, but they likely will in time. Even if they don't, you'll feel good about doing your part to help protect the future of our food and our planet.

Deal with Your Feelings About Going Against GMOs

It's amazing how something so basic as changing what you eat to more real food can evoke so many different feelings. There can be extreme anger (about the genetic hijacking of our food without our knowledge or consent), frustration (about how difficult it is to avoid GMOs), sorrow (for giving up foods you have fond memories of), and resentment (because avoiding GM foods is much more difficult compared to eating without thinking about what you're eating).

If you feel upset about many foods not being *food* anymore and about what an inconvenience it is to find real food, know that everyone who learns the real scoop about GMOs feels this way. Consider this Facebook conversation that took place between two people on exactly this subject:

> One woman wrote:

> *This whole issue of GMOs hidden in our food makes me sick to my core. I remember when we simply "ate food," which meant unadulterated nutrition for the human body. Now we have to go on a "hunt" to find wholesome fuel much like our first ancestors.*

> A man replied:

> *I hear you. Trying to buy healthy food at the grocery store for the kids is like a recon mission in enemy territory!*

If you experience these uncomfortable feelings, know that they're natural and that understanding this inconvenient truth is half the battle: It's what spurs people on to shop non-GMO and use our consumer power constructively.

To be most successful saying no to GMOs on a consistent basis, shift your thinking from focusing on the negative to the positive. Know that in the world of *real* food, there are still far more foods that are non-GMO than those that are genetically engineered. Focus on eating unadulterated whole foods like our ancestors did and make exploring healthy non-GMO foods you haven't tried before an exciting adventure.

Seek Support From Others

Don't go non-GMO alone, if at all possible. Look for understanding from friends and family members. If they aren't supportive, use this experience to speak from the heart and tell them why going non-GMO is important to you. You might be surprised that you'll get not only support but likely admiration and other people wanting to learn more and perhaps join in eating non-GMO.

Another way to seek out emotional (and practical) support is to join a non-GMO activist group, an Internet chat group, or a holistic parents group focused on this issue, such as Moms Across America. Finding others who feel like you do about the GMO issue—others with whom you can share your feelings, news, and tips—is exceptionally helpful in sticking with eating non-GMO over the long term.

Take An Occasional Short Break If You Need It

Although I recommend avoiding GMOs as much as possible, let me give you this heads-up: If you understand the urgency of the GMO situation and are strict about avoiding GMOs, you sometimes may get burnt out. Keeping up the intensity of avoiding GM foods against constant pressure from advertisements, television shows, and friends and acquaintances to eat typical American foods can get heavy and burdensome. (Sometimes you just want to beam yourself out of this food reality and have food be *real* food like it used to be!)

If you find yourself emotionally and spiritually drained from what seem like Herculean efforts you sometimes have to go through to avoid GM foods, give yourself a break once in a while. For example, relax in a restaurant and refrain from asking about minor sources of hidden GMOs, such as an oil in a salad dressing on an otherwise healthy salad, or just go out and have a dinner and a glass of wine with no questions asked. Having a few hours break from the constant effort it takes to avoid all sources of GMOs can do a world of wonders to relieve the stress that comes with maintaining such a huge effort. Also try non-food stress relievers: taking relaxing baths; listening to soothing music; and communing with nature. A bit of time to pull away from the situation allows you to recharge and come back all the stronger in your non-GMO effort.

LEARN NEW, PRACTICAL SKILLS

There's no getting around it: To consistently go against GMOs, you have to learn non-GMO skills to replace old food-preparation and eating habits. Then practice those skills until they become second nature.

The next several chapters will guide you through many different details of taking GMOs out of your diet. Here are some general guidelines to keep in mind:

1. Plan ahead.

This is rule number one for saying no to GM foods. Most of the commercial convenience foods sold in grocery stores contain genetically modified ingredients, so you can't just grab any food on the spur of the moment. You have to give more thought to what you're going to eat, and then prepare. Have ready-to-eat vegetables and fruits and other non-GMO snack foods at home. Get into the habit of carrying raw or dry-roasted nuts to eat. Keep your refrigerator and freezer well stocked with non-GMO foods, and set aside enough time in your schedule to prepare these foods.

2. Eat enough food and particularly enough protein.

Many of the most common sources of GMOs are processed convenience foods made from refined grains and sugars. If you avoid foods that contain hidden GM ingredients and experience strong cravings for grains and sugars, it's likely you're experiencing withdrawal symptoms from no longer eating regular amounts of those blood-sugar-spiking foods. You probably aren't eating enough protein, especially at breakfast. Eating enough protein is the most common dietary solution for controlling cravings and keeping energy levels steady to avoid grabbing quick-fix foods without thought and more easily stick with a non-GMO diet.

3. Keep GM foods out of your house and always have nutritious substitute foods on hand.

The easiest way to avoid GM foods is to not buy them or have ready access to them. Using non-GMO substitutes—i.e., eating non-GMO or organic corn chips in place of conventional corn chips—is a common technique that can be used to transition to a non-GMO diet. But it's important not to overdo these not-so-nutritious, non-GMO substitutes, as you'll learn in Chapter 8. It's far better to stock healthy, ready-to-eat, non-GMO whole foods, such as hard-boiled organic eggs, cooked organic meats, raw or dry-roasted nuts, unsweetened nut butter, and veggie sticks, which provide longer-burning fuel.

4. Keep meal preparation simple.

When you avoid GM foods the right way—by eating more whole foods—food preparation becomes less involved. Plus, the meals become more healing. Steer away from complicated recipes that contain a dozen or more ingredients. By using just a few fresh or seasonal foods and no processed foods, easy, uncomplicated dishes take on the taste of gourmet. For example, sprinkling herbs and olive oil or coconut oil over wild-caught fish and placing it in the oven doesn't take a lot of time but the end result is extremely tasty. By sautéing a big serving of vegetables in olive oil, you have yourself a meal.

5. Purposely make leftovers and look for other non-GMO shortcuts.

Make more non-GMO food than you plan to eat in one sitting. This tried-but-true technique lets you have reheated, healthy, fast food later in the week. Other helpful non-GMO shortcuts when you don't have time to cook include buying organic rotisserie chicken that you can eat off for a few meals and purchasing prepackaged, pre-washed salad mixes, veggie sticks, or cut-up vegetables from a natural food store salad bar.

6. Take the Eat GMO-Free Challenge in Chapter 7.

No matter what type of diet you eat, make the commitment to follow the Eat GMO-Free Challenge so you can learn the nitty-gritty details of how to remove GMO food impostors from what you eat. By learning a new tip each day for 31 days, you'll get a crash course on how to take the most common sources of GMOs out of your diet and grasp key non-GMO shopping and eating skills over the course of just one month.

Before moving onto the challenge, make sure to learn the four main guidelines for avoiding genetically engineered foods when making all food decisions. Those guidelines are up next.

Chapter 6:

Basic Going Against GMOs Eating Guidelines

Saying no to GMOs in the foods you buy and eat boils down to following only four guidelines. The principles are simple to understand and sound easy to follow. However, putting them into practice on a day-to-day basis takes time, as you'll understand in the next chapter.

Learn the following four guidelines and get them firmly cemented in your mind. After reading them several times, test yourself to see if you remember them when they aren't listed right in front of you. These strategies should be your guiding principles when making all food decisions, whether you're shopping in supermarkets, natural food stores, or farmers' markets, or eating out in restaurants.

GUIDELINE 1: BUY ORGANIC

Look for products with the USDA Organic seal, which means it's 100% organic or more than 95% organic. GMOs are an excluded ingredient in organic foods. In other words, certified organic products cannot intentionally include any GMO ingredients. For extra insurance, especially with foods that contain at-risk ingredients (listed in Guideline #3), look for products that have both the USDA Organic label *and* the Non-GMO Project Verified label.

GUIDELINE 2: LOOK FOR NON-GMO PROJECT SEALS

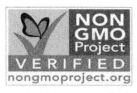

Choose products that carry the Non-GMO Project Seal. They are independently verified to be in compliance with North America's only third party standard for GMO avoidance, including testing of at-risk ingredients.

GUIDELINE 3: LEARN & AVOID THE 11 AT-RISK FOODS

Get the nine currently commercialized GM food crops firmly in your mind. Avoid foods that contain these common *direct food sources of GMOs* unless they are labeled organic or verified non-GMO. If you can't steer clear of all these foods in the beginning, focus on avoiding the first five, which are not healthy foods in general, as you'll learn in Chapter 8. One easy way to remember the at-risk crops is to keep this in mind: 3 Cs, 2 Ss, an A, a P, and a Y and a Z. The GM crops that are commercialized and now in our foods are:

- **Corn** (as in corn oil, cornmeal, cornstarch, corn syrup, hominy, polenta, and other corn-based ingredients)

- **Canola** (as in canola oil)

- **Cottonseed** (as in cottonseed oil)

- **Sugar Beets** (as in "sugar" in an ingredient, which is almost certainly a combination of sugar from both sugar cane and GM sugar beets—and also in foods that contain beet sugar)

- **Soybeans** (as in soybean oil, soy protein, soy lecithin, soy milk, tofu, and other soy-based ingredients)

- **Alfalfa** (which is fed to livestock)

- **Papaya** (from Hawaii and China)

- **Yellow Squash and Zucchini** (look for those labeled organic or grown from non-GMO seed)

Also avoid these two additional direct GM products that are added to foods:

- **Aspartame** (in diet soda and NutraSweet artificial sweetener)

- **rBGH** (recombinant Bovine Growth Hormone, also known as Bovine Somatotropin or BST.) It was developed from genetically engineered *E. coli* bacteria and is injected into some cows to increase milk production. Look for dairy products labeled rBGH-free, also known as BST-free, or better yet, for milk products labeled organic.

GUIDELINE 4: GRADUALLY UPGRADE THE ANIMAL PROTEIN SOURCES YOU EAT

This is a more advanced principle. Most people simply can't enact this guideline when they are first learning how to avoid GMOs, and some may never get to it. If you can't, that's okay. Focus on the first three and follow my step-by-step Eat GMO-Free Challenge in the next chapter. I guarantee that if you follow the previous three guidelines and the tips in the challenge, you will experience better health and help contribute to a mass movement to kick GM foods out of our food system.

Once you have eliminated the 11 direct food sources of GMOs, gradually work on removing the *indirect sources of GMOs* from your diet. This means avoiding conventional meats and dairy products from animals or farmed fish fed GM foods. Switch to eating more wild-caught fish, organic eggs and poultry, and meat labeled organic and preferably organic and 100% grass-fed—or fish, poultry, eggs, and meat labeled Non-GMO Project Verified. Taking GM crops out of animal feed is largely regarded as step 2 of kicking GMOs out of our food supply.

Ready to put these guidelines into practice? Read on to follow my Eat GMO-Free Challenge in the next chapter. If you follow a tip a day, within a month you will have received a jump-start into learning how to be a savvy non-GMO consumer. You'll also be giving your diet a major upgrade, transitioning from more processed convenience products (like in the Standard American Diet or SAD) to fresher, health-supporting, whole foods (upon which all healing diets are based!).

Chapter 7:

The Eat GMO-Free Challenge:
31 Tips for 31 Days

This chapter lists my series of 31 tips to help you learn how to avoid GMOs in foods. In 2011, with the help of a few other non-GMO advocates, I wrote the tips to serve as an education tool for a non-GMO group in southern Arizona and have revised them a few different times to use in my own practice.

The tips were designed to help people on any diet, including those on a typical American diet, slowly learn how to *remove or avoid direct sources of GMOs*, meaning the nine genetically modified crops, the artificial sweetener Nutrasweet (aspartame), and recombinant Bovine Growth Hormone (rBGH) found in dairy products.

The challenge builds up to more advanced tips to help people gradually learn how to *remove or reduce indirect sources of GMOs*, such as meat, eggs, and milk from animals fed GMOs. There are also Extra Tips that provide helpful information you may not know about certain foods, Bonus Tips offering practical or nutrition information to help your health, and words of motivation.

Make the commitment to try the challenge for a month. It may seem daunting at first, particularly if you view all the tips at once. However, the challenge is not as difficult as it looks. Discipline yourself to read one tip a day. (Or visit the Eat GMO-Free Challenge page on my website at EatGMOFreeChallenge.com, and click to have it display only one tip each day.) The challenge is much easier to grasp and complete that way.

Start whenever you'd like, and follow the tips for 31 consecutive days to learn step by step how to become a savvy non-GMO consumer by saying no to GMOs in real-life, day-to-day living.

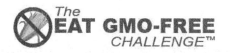

Tip #1

Freely eat all types of vegetables except for zucchini and yellow squash, a small amount of which is genetically modified. Seek out organic zucchini and yellow squash, or use Mexican grey squash in recipes that call for zucchini.

> **EXTRA TIP ABOUT VEGETABLES:** Most people think corn is a vegetable but it's really a grain. Genetically modified sweet corn started to appear in grocery stores in the autumn of 2011. Therefore, if you occasionally eat sweet corn, avoid it unless it's specifically labeled USDA organic or non-GMO or the farmer who grew it can assure you that it is from non-GMO sources.

Tip #2

Enjoy all types of fruit except papaya, especially papaya grown in Hawaii or China. (Genetically modified papayas are approved for cultivation in the United States and for consumption in the U.S. and Canada, but not in Europe. Unfortunately, most of the papaya now grown in Hawaii is genetically modified.)

> **BONUS TIP:** By "going against the grain" and eating more fresh vegetables and fruits instead of processed foods with grains and oils in them—as I wrote in my book *Going Against the Grain*—we automatically avoid most GMOs and eat a diet that is more health producing in numerous ways and that helps people lose weight when they need to. Think of all the foods you can enjoy without worry: cucumbers, leafy greens, celery, avocados, cabbage, peppers, onions, spinach, broccoli, asparagus, apples, pears, berries, and so many more!

Tip #3

Learn the 3 "C"s and 2 "S"s as a way to imprint the 5 major genetically modified crops in our food supply in your mind. The 3 "C"s are: Corn, Canola, and Cottonseed. The 2 "S"s are Soybeans, and Sugar from sugar beets. More detail about each of these foods will be covered in the next five tips and in Chapter 8.

> **BONUS TIP:** Make "label reading" a habit so you become aware of what's in your food. If you have a spouse or young kids who go shopping with you, teach them to read ingredients so they become aware, too, and they can help you spot at-risk ingredients.

Tip #4

To avoid GM corn, read food product labels and avoid those with obvious corn-based ingredients by looking for ingredients that contain the words "corn" or "maize" in them. Common examples include: corn oil, corn syrup, high-fructose corn syrup, corn starch, corn meal, corn masa (as in tamales), and maize starch. Steer clear of sweet corn and all foods that contain corn-based ingredients (including corn tortillas, corn chips, polenta, and corn grits) unless they are labeled USDA Organic or Non-GMO Project Verified.

> **EXTRA TIP ABOUT CORN:** A remedy to the GMO problem with yellow corn is finding heirloom blue cornmeal from conservation organizations such as Native Seeds/ SEARCH. However, if you have wide-ranging health problems—or if you are overweight (as most Americans are)—the evidence really points to going further against the grain and avoiding all forms of corn, including blue corn and organic corn products to regain your health. You'll learn more about that in the next chapter.

Tip #5

To avoid GM canola, look for canola oil in lists of ingredients and avoid those that contain it unless it is labeled organic or Non-GMO Project Verified. Canola oil is found in a wide range of products, including pasta sauces, salad dressings, mayonnaise, snack foods, prepared foods, and frozen entrees.

Tip #6

To avoid GM cottonseed, look for cottonseed oil in food product ingredients and avoid those that contain it. Cottonseed oil is sometimes in roasted nuts, snack foods, bread, and certain canned fish items.

Tip #7

To avoid GM soy, look for food products that say: Contains Soy (it should be clearly listed because Soy is a common allergen); or look for obvious ingredients that contain the words "soy" in the food product's list of ingredients. Common examples of soy-based ingredients include: soy protein, soy flour, soy sauce, soybean oil, soy milk, and soy lecithin. Tofu, tempeh, and miso are other sources of soy. Steer clear of foods with all of these ingredients unless they are labeled USDA Organic or Non-GMO Project Verified.

EXTRA TIP ABOUT VEGETABLE OILS: Even if they are not genetically modified, there are other important health reasons to avoid foods made with corn oil, canola oil, cottonseed oil, and soybean oil. As a general rule, vegetable oils are sources of omega-6 polyunsaturated fatty acids, which contribute to inflammatory diseases, including obesity, cardiovascular disease, type 2 diabetes, and autoimmune diseases, when eaten in excess. Plus, the fats in vegetable oils also are very easily damaged by heat, so they should not be used in cooking. The next chapter will explain more about health troubles caused by canola, cottonseed, corn, and soy.

Tip #8

To avoid sugar from GM sugar beets, read food product labels and don't buy foods that contain "sugar" or "beet sugar" in lists of ingredients. When not specified as sugar from sugar cane, "Sugar" in a list of ingredients almost always means a combination of sugar from sugar cane (which isn't genetically modified) and sugar from sugar beets (which is genetically modified).

> **EXTRA TIP ABOUT SUGAR:** Eating sugar generally should be avoided for many other health reasons. Whether GMO or not, eating refined sugar and other concentrated sweeteners contributes to elevated blood glucose and insulin levels, which over time sets off a whole cascade of events that lead to weight gain, common heart-disease risk factors, prediabetes, and diabetes. To learn more about this, consider reading my previous books *Syndrome X* and *Going Against the Grain.*

Tip #9

Stay away from soft drinks—both regularly sweetened and artificially sweetened. Regular soft drinks are sweetened with high-fructose corn syrup or sugar, both of which are derived from common GM crops (corn and sugar beets). Other soft drinks and sweetened waters are sweetened with fructose, another product derived from corn. "Diet" or artificially sweetened soft drinks are sweetened with aspartame (also known as Equal, Nutrasweet, Spoonful, or AminoSweet), another genetically modified product.

> **BONUS TIP:** When you first start to realize how many foods and beverages GMOs are hidden in, it can feel overwhelming and intimidating. It's a difficult process to gradually reduce or remove GMOs in your diet because GMOs are in a lot of products! Don't get discouraged or beat yourself up or give up. If you feel overwhelmed, realize that this reaction is almost universal. Virtually everyone feels that way when beginning the process of going non-GMO. Just

stay resolved to keep at it and do the best you can today. I promise that it will get easier. When changing any longstanding habits, the more you stick with it, the easier it becomes.

Tip #10

Ditch plain sugar in baking, and use maple syrup, stevia, unrefined cane sugar, coconut sugar or coconut nectar in its place. These sweeteners don't contain GMOs.

> **EXTRA TIP ABOUT HONEY:** Honey is not genetically modified but it is sometimes contaminated with GM pollen from plants such as GM canola or corn. If you want to use honey in special desserts, seek out a Non-GMO Project Verified honey, such as Wholesome Sweeteners Organic Amber Honey, Wedderspoon raw and organic honeys from New Zealand, or Rigoni di Asiago Mielbo Italian Honey.

Tip #11

Avoid processed foods and convenience foods as much as possible. Because almost all conventional corn, soy, and sugar beets grown in this county are genetically modified and subsidized by our government, they are cheap and end up in about 75 to 80 percent of processed foods in different forms.

Tip #12

Eat without worry all raw or dry-roasted nuts and seeds (without risky oils), all legumes except for soybeans, and organic or non-GMO unrefined grains such as Lotus Foods heirloom rice, Lundberg Farms brown rice, and Eden Foods quinoa or wild rice.

Tip #13

Avoid eating bread. If you eat bread, buy only Non-GMO Project Verified or USDA Organic bread, or try baking your own with non-GMO ingredients. In terms of GMOs, most breads available at grocery store chains contain multiple genetically modified ingredients including: high-fructose corn syrup; sugar; soy flour; soy oil; canola oil; cottonseed oil; and other soy and corn derivatives. Gluten-free bread often contains cornstarch, dextrose, fructose, and/or xanthan gum (all from GM corn) and often a genetically modified oil, such as canola, corn, or soybean oil.

> **BONUS TIP:** On your refrigerator, put up a Post-It note to keep reminding yourself why you're participating in the Eat GMO-Free Challenge. The note might say: *I am taking back my right for pure food*—or anything that keeps you strong and motivated. Also keep reading information about GMOs and sign up for newsletters from non-GMO educational organizations to stay educated. Keeping the information fresh in your mind about why it's important to continue staying away from GMOs is a very important part of sticking with eating non-GMO.

Tip #14

Cook with unrefined extra virgin olive oil or coconut oil instead of conventional butter, canola oil, vegetable oil, corn oil, or soybean oil. Conventional butter can contain GMOs and the latter four oils almost always contain GMOs. If you want to cook with butter, buy organic butter, which is free of GMOs—preferably organic pasture-raised butter.

Tip #15

If you eat milk products such as cheese or cream, look for organic or "rBGH- and rBST-free" milk products. rBGH (recombinant bovine growth hormone) is a synthetic growth hormone developed from genetically engineered *E coli* bacteria. It is not approved for use in most other countries besides the United States because of the health conditions it creates in dairy cows and the resulting pus, antibiotic, and vaccine residues in milk.

Tip #16

If you treat yourself to chocolate on occasion, buy organic chocolate. Most conventional chocolate bars contain high-fructose corn syrup, "sugar" (which is almost always from a combination of non-GMO cane sugar and GMO beet sugar), milk (that could be from cows that were injected with a genetically modified growth hormone), and soy lecithin (which is almost always GMO unless labeled organic or non-GMO).

Tip #17

Be careful about what you drink. Besides soft drinks that likely contain GMOs (tip #9), so too do any type of commercial sweetened beverage, including sweetened iced tea, and hot tea or coffee drinks such as lattes. To keep GMOs out of the beverages you drink, choose water, sparkling water (plain or with fruit essence), unsweetened iced tea, and coffee, tea or herbal tea (plain or sweetened at home with non-sugar sweeteners). To make a latte-type drink, use organic half-n-half or unsweetened canned coconut milk.

> **BONUS TIP:** Buy organic items when possible. Certified Organic products cannot intentionally contain GMOs. They are grown according to guidelines in which GMOs or toxic pesticides cannot be used, so eating organic foods offers health protection in many ways. Fortunately, it's easier than ever to buy organic items for often the same price or even lower than the price of conventional items. To get organic items affordably, watch the weekly grocery store ads carefully for organic items on sale, purchase local produce grown without pesticides at farmers' markets around town, or grow some of your own organic vegetables. When you can't buy organic, make sure to buy non-GMO conventional items.

Tip #18

For parties or snacking, buy corn chips that have the USDA organic seal or the Non-GMO Project Verified seal on them. For extra insurance, choose those that have both seals. RW Garcia (which is also gluten-free certified), the 365 brand, and Cadia are three companies to look for. For even more insurance against GMOs, choose blue corn chips with both seals on them. Blue corn is not genetically modified but most yellow corn and some types of white corn are.

Tip #19

To avoid corn-based chips altogether, purchase Non-GMO Project Verified bean-and-rice chips, such as those by Beanfields or Beanitos, rice chips or rice crackers such as those by Lundberg Farms, Edward & Sons, or Mary's Gone Crackers, or flaxseed-based snack foods, such as Flax Snax by Go Raw or Flax Crackers by Foods Alive. These products often can be found or special-ordered in natural food stores.

> **BONUS TIP:** Shop at your local health food store, which will contain many GMO-free alternatives that you won't find in regular grocery stores.

Tip #20

Take a zip-lock bag with your own organic chips to restaurants or events where you know that non-organic corn chips will be served. Keep in mind that more than 85 percent of corn grown in the United States is genetically modified, so it's important to eat only organic or Non-GMO Project Verified chips. Especially if you're going to a Mexican restaurant, bring your own chips and tell the waiter why you're doing so. If enough people speak up and say they're eating non-GMO, restaurants will make the switch to non-GMO chips.

A WORD OF MOTIVATION: Congratulations! You've made it three-quarters of the way through the Eat GMO-Free Challenge and have learned all the basics of how to eat GMO free. Way to go! Now keep going...

Tip #21

If you fall off the non-GMO wagon and eat a food that you know or think contains GMOs, don't be hard on yourself. Let it go, and get back on the non-GMO bandwagon as quickly as you can. It's not helpful to berate yourself for any "mistakes" you may have made with your diet. In learning to eat GMO free, we all have made mistakes, but those mistakes help us learn to be savvier consumers. Just get back on the Eat GMO-Free Challenge as quickly as possible. Doing so will protect your health from serious risks and play a part in creating the healthier food system we all want and deserve.

Tip #22

When you eat out, look for restaurants that cook exclusively with 100% pure olive oil (and that don't use vegetable oil, canola oil, corn oil, cottonseed oil, or soybean oil). That means mainly Greek, Italian, and Middle Eastern restaurants.

BONUS TIP: Inquire at restaurants, especially locally owned restaurants, about ingredients in the foods on their menus. Even when restaurants do not post labels for organic or GMO-free products, if you ask about ingredients and tell restaurant personnel that you avoid GMOs, you'll raise their awareness about the issue. It is surprising how many restaurant chefs do not know about GM foods. However, once they hear about them, they don't like the idea—and chefs and owners of locally run restaurants often can make changes on their menus quickly compared to those at chain restaurants.

Tip #23

When eating at restaurants, order items that do not contain any "at-risk" ingredients such as corn or soy unless they are organic. Common corn-based items on restaurant menus are corn tortillas, tamales, enchiladas, and tacos, and soy-based items include tofu, tempeh, miso, and soy sauce.

Tip #24

Choose salads as a relatively safe food choice to order in restaurants, as long as the salads don't contain at-risk foods, such as corn, corn tortilla strips, and soy sauce or vegetable oils in the salad dressing. Specifically ask what type of oil is in the salad dressings, and if they say "vegetable oil" or one of the four oils derived from GM foods (see tips 4-7), ask them if they can bring you 100% pure olive oil (not an olive oil/vegetable oil blend) and lemon or red wine vinegar to use on your salad.

Tip #25

Seek out restaurants with organic choices. Buying organic items is rule number one to safeguard against eating GMOs. Do not assume, though, that if a restaurant has "Organic" in its name that every item on its menu is organic. Always ask about at-risk ingredients such as corn to be sure.

> **BONUS TIP:** Speak to the managers or owners of your favorite restaurants and tell them how important it is to you that they have GMO-free and organic options. When enough people speak up, that sends the message loudly and clearly to restaurant managers and owners that there is a high demand for non-GMO, organic *real* food in restaurant meals. Furthermore, how we spend our money speaks volumes. When enough of us vote with our dollars by buying non-GMO meals, restaurants will get the message and begin offering more non-GMO and organic options on their menus.

Tip #26

Purchase Non-GMO Project Verified eggs or organic pastured eggs (from chickens that are not fed corn or soy that has been genetically engineered).

Tip #27

Switch to eating more and more organic and grass-fed meats and wild-caught fish and seafood. Conventionally raised animals are usually fed GMO corn and GMO soy-based diets, and farm-raised fish are often fed GMO feed, too. Organic and grass-fed meat and wild-caught fish are the way our sources of animal protein were until 70 years ago or so. Find local grass-fed meats at your local farmers' market. You can also purchase organic grass-fed meat and wild-caught fish at good sale prices periodically at natural food stores.

Tip #28

Enjoy a 100% grass-fed burger (without the bun) or a piece of wild-caught fish cooked in olive oil in a restaurant. Grass-fed burgers and wild-caught fish are two increasingly popular protein sources that are offered on some restaurant menus.

Tip #29

Read labels very carefully and check out the list in Appendix A to avoid "hidden" GMO ingredients. Common hidden forms of GMOs that are surprising to many people include xanthan gum, vitamin C, vitamin E, maltodextrin, and soy lecithin.

> **BONUS TIP:** Download the Non-GMO Shopping Guide app to your iPhone or the True Food Shoppers Guide mobile app for iPhone and Android—or the PDF guides to your computer—to help you do your shopping. For more info, see NonGMOShoppingGuide.com and CenterforFoodSafety.org.

Tip #30

Grow your own organic food, or buy organic food from a trusted source, and make more of your meals at home. This is the only way you can be completely sure that your meal is GMO free.

Tip #31

Keep reading information about GMOs to stay educated. Sign up for my *Against the Grain Nutrition News & Notes* e-newsletter and check out these other sites of good information about GMOs: the Institute for Responsible Technology, Organic Consumers Association, Food Democracy Now, GM Watch, and The Organic & Non-GMO Report. Keeping the information fresh in your mind is a very important part of sticking with eating non-GMO, and finding friends who are fellow non-GMO eaters is even better.

FINAL WORDS ABOUT THE CHALLENGE

Once you have completed the challenge, let me be the first to congratulate you on completing it! I bet you already feel better!

Remind yourself that you have protected your health from unknown risks of GMOs and have contributed to a collective movement to create positive change in our food system.

With fresher, less processed, real foods in your diet, you're bound to be healthier in the long run. So, don't stop. Keep it up and keep going…

Chapter 8:

Going Against GMOs for Optimal Health
Eating Guidelines

Now that you've learned the main foods in which GMOs tend to hide and the details of removing them from your diet, it's time to expand your nutrition knowledge to think beyond just non-GMO. Although avoiding GMOs is a key factor in making food your best medicine—so important that I made it the focus of this book—it is not, by any means, the only food factor necessary for creating and maintaining long-term health.

If you focus on eating non-GMO and nothing else, you'll likely develop health problems that don't have anything to do with GMOs. That statement may come as a surprise to many non-GMO advocates but unfortunately that's what I as a nutritionist see happening more and more often. You may not have realized this before, but *many foods that are labeled non-GMO are non-GMO junk foods that set us up for disease.* They may contain non-GMO versions of sugar, corn, soy, and canola oil, but those foods, whether GMO or not, are cheap filler foods that fatten people and contribute to disease over the long term.

As the first nutritionist to write a full-length book about non-GMO eating, I feel a responsibility to provide comprehensive nutrition information to prevent people from making dietary mistakes and developing unwanted ailments. I don't want the non-GMO movement to get derailed by people who don't understand important aspects of nutrition saying "non-GMO diets don't work." Toward those goals, this chapter gives a rundown of six eating guidelines to protect health, based on information covered in my previous books and my more than 20 years of experience counseling clients and doing in-depth study in nutrition.

It's important to understand the big picture of what we know about nutrition for optimal health because what's happening in the non-GMO movement right now is quite similar to what happened in the gluten-free movement. As more people learned about the health problems associated with gluten and realized they didn't want to eat it, they focused on avoiding gluten and nothing else. They ended up eating gluten-free foods—such as GMO corn, soy, and sugar, and refined white rice flour—that caused health problems for them in non-gluten ways. Now in the midst of the fast-growing non-GMO movement, many people are laser-focused on avoiding GMOs. *However, I see them making nutritional mistakes eating non-GMO foods that promote health problems in non-GMO-related ways.*

The typical advice to eat non-GMO, as I covered in Chapter 6, is to avoid the top GM products, unless they are labeled non-GMO or organic. But we need to go further. The nutrition guidelines we individually need to promote health are also what we collectively need to pursue to change our agriculture system away from producing outrageous amounts of unhealthy foods. The way to do that is to go further against the status quo by avoiding even non-GMO or organic forms of the Big Five GM foods and other highly subsidized foods, such as wheat, that derail health.

GOING AGAINST GMOs FOR OPTIMUM HEALTH EATING GUIDELINES

1. Avoid sugar and other sweeteners (whether GMO or not).

2. Ditch artificial sweeteners (whether GMO or not).

3. Go against the grain: Eat more non-starchy vegetables, and avoid wheat & gluten.

4. Be wary of corn, soy, or milk products (whether GMO or not).

5. Steer clear of vegetable oils and trans-fats (whether GMO or not).

6. Limit exposure to chemicals, including pesticides and food additives, and eat as "clean" a diet as possible.

It's time to expand on what you learned in Chapters 6 and 7 about how to say no to GMOs and add to it by learning how to avoid other problematic ingredients associated with disease. Above I have listed six guidelines for designing a non-GMO diet for optimal health. I'll start now explaining each one in greater detail.

Guideline 1: Avoid Sugar & Sweeteners (Whether GMO or Not)

Many people who are aware of the health problems associated with GMOs are avoiding GM beet sugar but freely purchasing and eating foods made with cane sugar, often called evaporated cane juice, which is not presently genetically engineered in the United States. Doing that is a mistake. Although avoiding GMOs is always better than not avoiding them, it's absolutely essential to understand that sugar, whether GMO or not, is hazardous to our health in the following ways:

- Sugar puts people on a blood sugar roller coaster where blood sugar—and energy and mood levels—spike, then crash.

- Sugar suppresses immune function: It reduces the ability of white blood cells to track and attack bacteria and also reduces the production of antibodies, which protect against viruses and other invaders.

- Sugar feeds yeast and unbeneficial bacteria, which promote yeast overgrowth and harmful bacterial overgrowth in the gut that lead to conditions such as gas and bloating.

- Sugar overconsumption leads to high blood glucose and high blood insulin levels that set off a cascade of metabolic events, which over time promote accelerated aging and the development of numerous degenerative diseases, including cardiovascular disease and type 2 diabetes. (You can learn more about this in my book *Syndrome X*.)

Sugar overconsumption is now regarded as an independent risk factor in cardiovascular disease, which includes heart attacks, strokes, and artery disease, as well as type 2 diabetes, liver cirrhosis, and dementia. These diseases are all linked to metabolic syndrome (or Syndrome X), which involves unhealthy blood fat levels, hypertension, and insulin resistance.[131] One 2014 study found that compared with people who consumed less than 10 percent of calories from added sugar, people who ate between 10 and 25 percent of their calories from added sugar were 30 percent more likely to die of cardiovascular disease.[132] This applies to most of the American population: About 71 percent of U.S. adults consume more than 10 percent of their calories from added sugar.

Sugar also has become a major focus in cancer research: Researchers have found that high levels of insulin produced by the body in response to eating or drinking sugar drive the growth of many cancers.[133] A segment on *60 Minutes* interviewed key scientists conducting these newer studies who said they have been so influenced by what they found that they changed their own eating habits to avoid sugar.[134]

All this research points to this: *For optimal health, avoid eating sugar on a regular basis.* The best policy is to remove from your diet all sweetened foods, beverages including fruit juice, concentrated sweeteners of any type, and flour products, such as bread, that quickly convert to sugars, so your blood sugar metabolism and overall health can recover and normalize. Sure, when you first eliminate sugar, you're likely to experience withdrawal symptoms, such as cravings or irritability. But if you're on the right diet—meaning a blood-sugar-balancing diet— the unpleasant symptoms typically disappear or greatly diminish after the better part of a week, and mood and energy levels improve. You'll also automatically start to lose excess weight and experience dramatic improvements in blood sugar levels and other heart-disease risk factors.

DIFFERENT FORMS OF SUGAR TO AVOID

Though some of the following may sound healthy and some may not, and some are derived from GM foods and some are not, all of them mean sugar, which wreaks havoc on the body. Steer clear of all of them.

Barley malt	High-fructose corn syrup
Beet sugar	Honey
Blackstrap molasses	Malt syrup
Brown sugar	Maltodextrin
Cane juice crystals	Maple sugar
Cane sugar	Maple syrup
Confectioner's sugar	Molasses
Corn syrup	Raw sugar
Dextrose	Rice Syrup
Evaporated cane juice	Sucrose
Fructose	Sugar
Fruit juice	Syrup
Fruit juice concentrate	Turbinado sugar

GUIDELINE 2: DITCH ARTIFICIAL SWEETENERS (WHETHER GMO OR NOT)

Except for the fact that genetically modified foods are not labeled and artificial sweeteners are, the situation with artificial sweeteners is similar to the situation with GM foods. Artificial sweeteners, such as aspartame (Nutrasweet), saccharin (SweetNLow), and sucralose (Splenda), are, well, *artificial*. That already should tell you something. They are created in a laboratory for the benefit of the companies that make them, are not safe, and should have never been allowed on the market. Yet they have been allowed into our food supply for decades because of deception by big business and governmental agencies (that sounds familiar, doesn't it?) and many people assume they're safe because they're found in grocery stores and restaurants.

ARTIFICIAL SWEETENERS TO AVOID

Acesulfame potassium   Saccharin (SweetNLow)
Aspartame (NutraSweet)   Sucralose (Splenda)
Cyclamate

Do your body a favor and stay away from unnatural sugar substitutes. Aspartame is a genetically modified product and it may be the worst of the bunch, but make no mistake about it: None of the artificial sweeteners are good for you. Taken all together, the different artificial sweeteners have been linked to a whopping list of problems, including cancers (such as leukemia and non-Hodgkin's lymphoma), migraines, depression, dizziness, neurological conditions, seizures, behavior changes, anemia, and thyroid dysfunction.

From my experience counseling clients, consuming foods or drinks with artificial sweeteners, such as diet soda, perpetuates the need for the sweet taste, and keeps people craving, wanting, and having more and more "sweet stuff." I have found it impossible to get people to stop craving and eating sugar when they use artificial sweeteners.

Experiments have found that the sweet taste, regardless of its caloric content, enhances a person's appetite. Artificial sweeteners also might cause a phenomenon called calorie dysregulation where the body gets confused from the lack of calories that go with that sweet taste. The body expects sugar and prepares for sugar, but there is none; so it compensates, craving the calories it was primed for and throwing the system off balance.

Also, since artificial sweeteners are many times sweeter than sugar, they modify our experience of sweetness, meaning we need more and sweeter things to satisfy cravings. Far from helping people lose weight, they may actually promote weight gain more than sugar.

If you've been regularly using aspartame or other artificial sweeteners, I recommend getting off them as soon as possible. Beware, though: Cutting them from your diet may lead to withdrawal symptoms, such as on-and-off headaches, nausea, or cravings for sweets, which can sometimes last two weeks to a month. If you experience uncomfortable symptoms, recognize these as clear indications of the dysfunction and ill health that artificial sweeteners have been causing and know you're doing the body good to eliminate them.

GUIDELINE 3: GO AGAINST THE GRAIN: EAT MORE NON-STARCHY VEGETABLES, AND AVOID WHEAT & GLUTEN

Going against the grain—cutting the excessive grains people eat and replacing them with non-starchy vegetables—has been the central focus of my work with clients for more than a decade. On the most basic level, grains and grain-based products, such as wheat flour and rice flour, are high in calories and blood-sugar-spiking carbohydrates and relatively low in nutrients compared to the calories they provide. Grain-based convenience foods, such as breads, crackers, pizza, and baked goods, also are some of the most common sources of hidden GM ingredients, such as sugar, fructose, high-fructose corn syrup, corn oil, soy protein, soybean oil, and canola oil. For these reasons, avoiding high-carb, high-calorie grain products and replacing them with more low-carb, low-calorie vegetables is an important food strategy that can benefit all of us.

Non-starchy vegetables (those that aren't root vegetables such as potatoes or winter squash) are the types of carbohydrates humans evolved on and are designed to thrive on. The more vegetables we eat, the better it is for protecting health and preventing disease. One 2014 study in the *Journal of Epidemiology and Community Health* concluded that each daily portion of fresh vegetables reduces the overall risk of death by 16 percent![135] Yet study after study shows that many Americans eat a paltry amount of vegetables. *When people eat more vegetables in place of grains, they dramatically, effortlessly lose unwanted weight, improve their health in many different ways, and recover from countless conditions, such as autoimmune conditions, type 2 diabetes, prediabetes, and common heart-disease risk factors, including abdominal fat, high blood pressure, and high triglycerides.*

NON-STARCHY VEGETABLES — THE ONES TO EMPHASIZE

All lettuces and greens	Green, red & Chinese cabbage
Asparagus	Mushrooms
Bok choy	Spinach
Broccoli	Sweet and hot peppers
Cauliflower	Yellow wax beans and green beans
Celery	Zucchini and yellow summer squash (choose organic or heirloom summer squash)
Cucumber	

A crucial part of going against the grain for optimal health is avoiding wheat and gluten. (Gluten is the problematic protein in wheat, rye, barley, and most oats.) As I described in my previous book *Going Against the Grain*, wheat is high glycemic, and high in carbohydrates, lectins (such as wheat germ agglutinin, which increases gut permeability and causes an unhealthy imbalance in gut bacteria), and antinutrients (such as phytate that blocks the absorption of key minerals in the body and leads to a host of health problems resulting from nutrient deficiencies). Many people aren't aware that high-wheat diets are implicated in most modern-day health problems—everything from bone diseases, such as osteoporosis, to autoimmune diseases, such as autoimmune thyroid disease, to the major killers of today, such as type 2 diabetes and heart disease.

Unfortunately, the toxic health effects from wheat and gluten have become even worse this century because of newfangled agriculture techniques—hybridization, backcrossing, and inducing mutations through the use of chemicals—that have been performed on wheat in an effort to increase yield. Although hybridized wheat was assumed safe, no safety studies were ever done on it (which was very similar to what happened with genetically modified foods), and that was unfortunate: We now know that wheat gluten proteins, in particular, undergo considerable structural change with hybridization. In one hybridization experiment, 14 new gluten proteins were identified! The incidences of the autoimmune disease associated with gluten intake, celiac disease, and non-celiac gluten sensitivity are both on the rise—and those conditions are associated with more than 200 different health conditions.

There's now a wealth of several hundred clinical studies on adverse and sometimes crippling effects of wheat consumption in humans—way more than there were when I wrote *Going Against the Grain* in 2002. The studies, many of which are written about in *Wheat Belly* by cardiologist William Davis, M.D., document neurologic impairments unique to wheat, including cerebellar ataxia and dementia; heart disease; visceral fat accumulation and all its many health consequences; and the process of glycation (via the blood-sugar-spiking carbohydrate, amylopectin A, in wheat) that leads to cataracts, diabetes, and arthritis. In a nutshell, if you say goodbye to wheat and gluten, and eat more vegetables, you say goodbye to more health problems and diseases than you can imagine.

As a final note in this guideline, let me clear up a common misconception: Genetically modified wheat is not yet on the market. Although it has been developed, has been planted in test plots around the United States, and apparently has contaminated at least one commercial wheat plot in Oregon, GM wheat has not yet been commercialized. Rather, the ill health effects from wheat stem from our bodies not being designed to properly digest wheat and function well on it in the first place, plus hybridization and other techniques used during the past 50 years or so, including spraying glyphosate herbicide just prior to harvest, that have dramatically changed wheat so that it has become even more toxic to us.

**COMMON SYMPTOMS ASSOCIATED
WITH GLUTEN SENSITIVITY**

The following, while not a complete list, is a list of some of the more common symptoms associated with gluten sensitivity.

Acid-reflux-type conditions

Anemia

Autoimmune diseases (including autoimmune thyroid disease, rheumatoid arthritis, and type 1 diabetes)

Depression

Bone disease (including osteopenia and osteoporosis)

Constipation and/or diarrhea

Fatigue and tiredness

Gas and bloating

Neurological conditions (including attention deficit hyperactivity disorder, headaches/migraines, and ataxia)

Skin conditions (including dermatitis herpetiformis, eczema and psoriasis)

Unexplained infertility

Source: *Gluten Free Throughout the Year*

GUIDELINE 4: BEWARE OF CORN, SOY, AND MILK PRODUCTS (WHETHER GMO OR NOT)

Corn, soy, cow's milk, and wheat (which was described in the previous guideline) are relatively new foods in the human diet. Humans did not originally evolve on these foods and we are not well adapted to them. Over time, we can develop numerous health issues from eating these foods, including food allergies and delayed-onset food sensitivities. Soy, milk, and wheat have long been known to be among the world's top food allergens. Plus, as I explained in Chapter 3, allergies to corn are now on the rise, and allergies to soy increased in England after GM soy was introduced there. Many non-GMO eaters have allergies to one or more of these foods.

THE TROUBLE WITH WHEAT, CORN, SOY, & MILK

- Wheat, corn, soy, and milk are foods to which we aren't well adapted
- They're heavily subsidized by the U.S. government and form major parts of the Standard American Diet (SAD)
- They cause health problems in many different ways over time and are common food allergens

---

Even if you aren't allergic to corn, soy, milk, or wheat, it's still important to avoid or greatly limit your intake of these foods because they're foods that make us sick over time. Unfortunately, the U.S. government heavily subsidizes the large-scale production of these foods, which has led to excessive amounts of them being added into countless foods. Both to protect our health and to change the system so our land can be used to produce more diversified and nutritious foods, we should go against these highly subsidized foods, whether they're GMO or not.

This guideline will cover the reasons to avoid non-GMO corn, soy, and milk. The next guideline will cover reasons to avoid non-GMO foods used to create vegetable oils.

If We Are What We Eat, Americans Are Corn and Soy

– Headline on a CNN Health article from Sept. 22, 2007

Corn

Whether it's genetically modified or not, corn is a high-carbohydrate, high-glycemic (or blood-sugar-spiking) food that fattens cattle and does the same to us when eaten in excess. With more than two-thirds of the population overweight, it's outrageous to have corn the most subsidized food by the U.S. government and produced in such enormous amounts that it is added to virtually all processed foods. Besides the fact that virtually all industrially produced corn is genetically modified, most of it is hybridized, too. It's possible that hybridization might have caused some unintended side effects in corn as it did with wheat.

As mentioned, allergies to corn are reported more and more often. People with corn allergies have become so sensitive that they typically need to avoid all forms of corn, including non-GMO, heirloom, and organic corn, to recover from wide-ranging symptoms. People who are overweight or have blood sugar- or insulin-related health problems do best lowering their blood sugar levels, losing weight, and recovering their health when they avoid all types of corn.

Even if you don't think you have health issues or don't think you eat much corn, you probably don't realize that our entire food supply has undergone a process that author Michael Pollan calls "cornification" in recent years, without our even noticing it. Cheap corn sweeteners, such as high-fructose corn syrup, are added into everyday foods by food manufacturers, and corn is now a primary ingredient in feed for factory-farmed chicken, pigs and cows and even for many farm-raised fish. Corn is used to make corn oil and partially hydrogenated corn oil, which are found in many snack foods, margarines and baked goods; to make high-fructose corn syrup, the most prevalent and cheapest of all sweeteners; and to make countless food additives.

To get an idea of how corn crazy our food supply is, go to the supermarket and read the label of virtually any mass-produced commercial food. You'll be hard-pressed to find one without corn of some type in its list of ingredients (except for commercial meat, which, of course, isn't labeled as such but is from animals fattened on corn nonetheless).

In fact, most of the corn produced in excessive amounts in this country is used for the completely unnatural process of feeding it to animals such as cows for industrial meat production instead of feeding cows grass as they were designed for. Only a tiny fraction of corn grown in the U.S. directly feeds the nation's people, and much of that is from high-fructose corn syrup!

Also, consider this: The production of corn requires more nitrogen fertilizer and more pesticide than any other crop, so growing literally mountains and mountains of corn pollutes U.S. rivers and soil, wreaking havoc on the environment. What's more, nitrogen fertilizer is made from natural gas, and pesticides are made from oil, so growing so much corn guzzles fossil fuel—something we definitely don't need in this age of rising gas prices.

Because our whole food supply system is centered around corn, the rising cost of corn spills over into the rising cost of foods across the board. As Jonathan Foley, director of the Institute on the Environment at the University of Minnesota, wrote in a 2013 article reprinted in *Scientific American*, the American corn system is inefficient at feeding the American people a more diverse and nutritious diet. Corn uses more land than any other U.S. crop and uses large amounts of other natural resources such as water, and it's highly vulnerable to disaster, disease, and pests, as are all massive monoculture agricultural systems.[136]

It's time to understand the American corn system has created a mess in more ways than one for us. If we take a stand and as much as possible avoid mass-produced sources of even non-GMO corn, including corn-fed meat sources, we emphatically say no to the corn-centered system that is making us sick.

Soy Foods

Soy isn't the health food many people now think it is. It actually went from being an unpopular food to being added to virtually all processed foods and consumers sometimes now seek out processed fake soy-based products like "soy milk." How did that happen? Food manufacturers intent on creating cheap vegetable oils convinced the U.S. government to start subsidizing the production of soy, and more of it started being grown at our expense as taxpayers. Soy was turned into an unhealthy oil, and the industry was left with industrial waste products, such as isolated soy protein, which the industry spun as healthy ingredients to eat.

Given all the hype you hear about soy, it may come as a surprise to you that soy on its own is an unhealthy food. Soy contains many health-disrupting antinutrients, including:

- **Phytates**, which block mineral absorption in the human digestive tract, causing zinc, iron and calcium deficiencies;

- **Lectins and saponins,** which are linked to 'leaky gut' and other gastrointestinal and immune system problems;

- **Goitrogens**, substances that block the synthesis of thyroid hormones and interfere with iodine metabolism, thereby disrupting thyroid function that is vital for a healthy metabolism;

- **Protease inhibitors, including trypsin inhibitors**, which reduce the body's ability to digest protein and can cause malnutrition, poor growth, and digestive distress.

In *The Whole Soy Story*, author Kaayla Daniel, Ph.D., C.C.N., summarizes thousands of studies linking soy to malnutrition, digestive distress, immune system breakdown, thyroid dysfunction, cognitive decline, reproductive disorders and infertility. Also, bear in mind that soy is a common allergen—it is one of the top eight food allergens in the world—and it can cause soy sensitivity or intolerance that is different from an allergy. Soy allergy symptoms include hives or other skin rashes, trouble breathing, abdominal pain or diarrhea, and nausea or vomiting. Symptoms of soy sensitivity are large amounts of intestinal gas, abdominal pain and cramps, and bloating of the belly.

Consider this: Soybeans were not considered fit for humans until the Chinese learned to ferment them into the forms of natto, miso, tamari, and tempeh. Fermentation reduces some of the main antinutrients in soy and makes it more digestible. Asian diets now include only about 2 *teaspoons* of soy a day, usually as a condiment, and it's highly fermented! Most of the soy products Americans are eating are not fermented, which means we're consuming all the antinutrients that come with non-fermented soy.

Sure, soy is *the* most genetically modified and heavily sprayed food. But for nutritional reasons that go far beyond those compelling factors, I recommend avoiding soy entirely. I don't believe we should support the large-scale farming of a food with so many nutritional problems associated with it. If you choose to use soy, I recommend that you seek out fermented, gluten-free, organic and Non-GMO Project Verified soy products, such as miso or tamari, and use them in minimal amounts as condiments.

Milk

Cow's milk was designed by nature to nourish baby cows, not us. But modern feeding methods of giving cows soy and corn instead of grass, breeding methods to increase milk production, and using antibiotics and sometimes genetically modified recombinant bovine growth hormone (rBGH) in dairy cattle have created cow's milk that is much more unnatural and unhealthy for us.

Just as our bodies don't tolerate gluten in wheat, our bodies have similar trouble handling certain proteins in milk, such as casein. *Cow's milk is the number one food allergen in this country*, and milk allergy contributes to gastrointestinal distress of all types, including diarrhea, cramps, bloating, gas, and gastrointestinal bleeding, and many cases of asthma, autism, bronchitis, iron-deficiency anemia, and skin rashes. Consuming milk products is the primary cause of recurrent ear infections in children. It also has been linked to insulin dependent diabetes and rheumatoid arthritis.

One aspect of dairy products that isn't well known is that *many dairy products, such as ice cream, cottage cheese, and even highly touted yogurt, have a high insulin index*: they induce a large quantity of the fat-storing hormone insulin in the blood after they are consumed—and preventing high insulin levels is important for preventing insulin-related degenerative diseases. Dairy products also contain opioids that set the stage for dairy cravings and addictions in some people.

Though milk is high in calcium, which is needed for healthy bones, most of us don't understand that calcium balance is far more important for bone health than calcium intake, and the acid-alkaline balance of the diet determines calcium balance. Dairy products as a group are acidic. When too many acidic foods in the diet are consumed, the body pulls calcium out of the bones to buffer the acidity. What this means is instead of loading up on milk products, a far more effective way to improve calcium balance and protect bone health is to eat more fresh vegetables and fruits! Researchers have found that those who eat the most fruits and vegetables have denser bones. Not only are fruits and vegetables rich in potassium, magnesium, calcium, and other nutrients essential for bone health, but researchers have concluded that because fruits and vegetables are alkaline, not acid-producing, they do not induce calcium loss in the urine.

Since sensitivity to milk products is exceedingly common, most of my clients experience their best health by not eating any dairy products or using them in limited amounts. If you don't have allergies and choose to eat dairy items, start with butter, preferably organic pasture-raised butter, the healthiest choice; use dairy items more as condiments; and select the highest quality milk products you can afford. Choose rBGH-free over conventional, USDA organic or Non-GMO Project Verified over rBGH-free, and preferably organic 100% pasture-raised (which are higher in healthy omega-3 fats) over just organic (which typically means from cows fed organic corn and soy).

GUIDELINE 5: STEER CLEAR OF REFINED VEGETABLE OILS & TRANS-FATS (WHETHER GMO OR NOT)

Many people perceive vegetable oils as healthy. Perhaps that is because the word "vegetable" is in the term, but vegetables don't have anything to do with them. Instead, four of the Big Five highly subsidized GM foods—corn, soy, cottonseed, and canola—are used to produce the most common refined vegetable oils. Safflower and sunflower seeds, which are not genetically modified, are other foods used to make vegetable oils. All are relatively new additions to the human diet. Unlike traditionally used oils such as olive or coconut oils, which can be easily pressed to create the oils, vegetable oils weren't eaten until the early 1900s when chemical processes allowed them to be extracted and produced on a large scale. Then they began to be eaten in high amounts in the 1960s and 1970s when government guidelines (unfortunately) advocated consuming them.

Just as eating refined sugar contributes to the development of disease over time, so too does eating refined vegetable oils, which are high in omega-6 fats. Our bodies need a balance of omega-6 fats and omega-3 fats. (Omega-3s are found in fatty fish and grass-fed meat and dairy products.) Both are essential fats needed for health. But over the last century, our diets have shifted almost completely to omega-6 fats primarily because we've been eating vegetable oils humans never ate before. *Too many omega-6 fats and too few omega-3 fats in the diet depress immune system function, and promote insulin resistance and inflammation in the body.* That applies to whether the vegetable oils are from GM sources (corn, soy, or cottonseed), non-GMO versions of those oils, or from non-GMO sources such as safflower or sunflower oils. Soybean oil is particularly problematic: It's hard to believe, but it's estimated that on average, 20 percent of all calories in the U.S. diet may come from soybean oil.

VEGETABLE OILS TO AVOID

Canola oil   Safflower oil
Corn oil   Sunflower oil
Cottonseed oil   Soybean oil
Partially hydrogenated oil
of any type

A few words about canola oil, which is used in most restaurants and found in countless products sold in natural food supermarkets: Canola oil is different from other vegetable oils because it is not especially high in omega-6 fats. It is highest in monounsaturated fats and also has some omega-3 fats—two reasons it is touted as "heart healthy." But it is a highly refined vegetable oil from a heavily sprayed, industrially produced crop. Just as other foods that aren't good for us have been pushed by the food industry into our food supply in high amounts, so, too, has canola oil.

Canola oil was developed by making a hybrid version of rape seed. (Rape seed oil contains high amounts of erucic acid, which is toxic to humans. So rape seed had to be hybridized to remove most of the erucic acid.) LEAR oil, which stands for Low Erucic Acid Rapeseed, was slow to catch on among consumers, so in the late 1970s, the industry renamed the product "canola" for "Canadian oil" because most of the new rape seed at the time was grown in Canada. Through a clever marketing and "education" campaign, the industry gradually convinced the public to believe canola oil was good for them and accept it as an oil to eat. Today, most of it is genetically modified and sprayed with excessive amounts of herbicide, and like all vegetable oils, canola oil is produced using unhealthy industrial production methods. A combination of high-temperature mechanical pressing and solvent extraction are used to remove the oil from the seeds, and traces of solvent, usually hexane, remain in the oil. The oil is then refined, bleached, and degummed—processes that involve high temperatures or chemicals of questionable safety. The omega-3 fatty acids that canola contains can easily become rancid or foul-smelling, so canola oil then must be deodorized, and deodorizing can turn some of the omega-3 fatty acids in it into unhealthy trans-fats.[137]

Consumer acceptance of canola oil represents one in a series of victories for the food processing industry, which has as its goal the replacement of all traditional foods with imitation foods made out of products derived from corn, wheat, soybeans, and oil seeds.

– Sally Fallon and Mary G. Enig, Ph.D., in their article, "The Great Con-ola"

Vegetable oils, such as canola oil and soybean oil, also are sometimes hydrogenated by forcing gas into the oils at high pressure. The completely unnatural man-made fats created through the partial hydrogenation process form trans-fats, which are used to make margarine, vegetable shortening, and oils that are used in high-temperature, deep-fat frying or added to processed foods such as cookies and crackers. Trans-fats cause dysfunction and chaos in the body on a cellular level—and they promote obesity and insulin resistance and *double the risk of heart disease.* Even though consumers have been gradually moving away from trans-fats over the past decade and fewer food companies are using them, as I explained in Chapter 3, the Centers for Disease Control and Prevention estimates that a further reduction of trans-fats in the food supply could prevent an additional 7,000 deaths from heart disease each year and up to 20,000 heart attacks each year.

Whether from GMO sources or not, vegetable oils and trans-fats are cheap, industry-created refined fats known to be major contributors to disease. It's extremely difficult to avoid convenience foods, such as salad dressings, sauces, and snack foods, that don't contain these oils, but the more you can avoid refined vegetable oils and trans-fats in all the foods you purchase, the healthier you will be.

Instead of newfangled vegetable oils, the best oils to use in food preparation at home are organic extra virgin olive oil and coconut oil. They have a long history of use among humans. Other fats to use on occasion include unrefined macadamia nut oil, sesame oil, and organic, preferably pasture-raised butter.

GUIDELINE 6: AVOID EXPOSURE TO CHEMICALS, INCLUDING PESTICIDES AND FOOD ADDITIVES, AND EAT AS "CLEAN" A DIET AS POSSIBLE

We tend to think food is pretty much the same as the organic *real* food our great grandparents ate. Most of us don't realize how chemically driven modern industrial food production has become. We also tend to assume that anything added to food today has been tested and found to be safe.

By reading this book, you know that there has been an explosion in the use of chemical herbicide sprayed on crops we use as foods. The most heavily used herbicide, Roundup, is sprayed on subsidized crops such as sugar, corn, soy, and wheat, and research links exposure to Roundup with increases in birth defects and some cancers. You also know that genetically engineered ingredients that are now in the majority of pro-cessed foods were never independently tested and found safe. They were essentially allowed on the market by the companies that made them. The same is true for chemical food additives used in factory-made foods.

Just as the FDA conducts no testing of its own on GM foods, it also does not conduct testing on thousands of food additives that have been added to our food supply in the past several decades. With the enactment of the Food Additives Amendment of 1958, Congress allowed a manufacturer or trade association to decide on its own that a chemical's use is generally recognized as safe, or allowed the manufacturer to petition the FDA or ask the FDA to review its safety decision for a chemical use. Even if the FDA raises concerns about that chemical, a manufacturer may withdraw its notification without penalty and is still able to use the chemical because the manufacturer deems it safe. Consequently, an astounding amount of manufacturer-driven food additives have been introduced into our food supply in recent decades. The Pew Charitable Trusts' Food Additives Project estimates that there are more than 10,000 chemicals allowed in food, and manufacturers or trade association panels approved more than 3,000 of these chemicals without any FDA review.[138]

Hazards to health from some food additives, such as artificial sweeteners and partially hydrogenated oil, have already been discussed earlier in this chapter. More than 100 food additives are usually derived from genetically modified ingredients, especially GM corn and soy, which are associated with numerous health problems including immune system and gastrointestinal problems. The majority of coloring additives used today are derived from coal tar and contain some carcinogens (cancer-causing substances). Some food additives cause other harmful effects, such as serious allergic reactions. Perhaps the most compelling reason to be concerned is nobody has ever tested the thousands of chemicals and food additives now used in food in combination with each other.

The United States has repeatedly taken the side of industry concerning use of genetically modified ingredients, food additives, and other chemical ingredients in our foods. In Europe and other parts of the world, they take a different approach, simply calling food "food" and clearly labeling foods that contain genetically engineered ingredients. People, therefore, have accurate information, and virtually no one buys them.

Europe has much stricter bans on food additives than the United States and, given the lack of long-term studies that have been conducted on food additives, it doesn't use ingredients like high-fructose corn syrup and genetically engineered ingredients. Europe also has higher standards for meat production than the United States: It doesn't allow antibiotics to be given to animals in "sub-therapeutic" amounts to make them gain weight as is common in this country.[139] Europe also doesn't use artificial growth hormones in meat production, and it so far has rejected imports of U.S.-raised beef from cattle raised with growth hormones.[140 141]

Though the President's Cancer Panel urges the public to reduce its exposure to the myriad of chemicals in our environment, our government agencies aren't enacting public policy to help us do that, so it's important for us to take action on our own and protect ourselves. In terms of reducing exposure to chemicals, food additives, and pesticides in food, try these tips:

- **Steer clear of the Big Five (sugar, soy, corn, canola, and cottonseed) + Wheat.** These foods are sprayed with dramatically increased levels of herbicide, especially Roundup.

- **Avoid processed foods with lists of ingredients that contain hard-to-pronounce words.** The unrecognizable ingredients are almost always derived from chemicals or industrially produced derivatives of subsidized foods that aren't good for us.

- **Eat organic foods as much as possible.** That's the easiest way to avoid GMOs and other nasty industrial agriculture ingredients, including synthetic chemical pesticides and fertilizers, sewage sludge, antibiotics, and artificial growth hormones.

REASONS TO CHOOSE ORGANIC

When you eat organic, you reduce your exposure to many different undesirable, artificial and chemical substances. Under the United States Department of Agriculture (USDA) National Organic Program, organically produced foods must be produced **without the use** of:

- Antibiotics (in the production of meat, dairy, and eggs)

- Artificial growth hormones (in the production of meat, dairy, and eggs)

- High-fructose corn syrup (because of the chemicals used in its production)

- Artificial dyes (made from coal tar and petrochemicals)

- Artificial sweeteners

- Synthetically created chemical pesticides and fertilizers

- Genetically modified ingredients (or GMOs)

- Sewage sludge (used as a fertilizer)

- Irradiation (which means applying ionizing radiation to food)

FINAL WORDS ABOUT EATING NON-GMO
FOR OPTIMAL HEALTH

In this chapter, I've gone beyond just non-GMO and covered the in-depth details of how laboratory created fake ingredients and foods to which we aren't well adapted are known contributors to disease. I hope by now you see the big picture that none of us should allow ourselves to be guinea pigs eating foreign or unknown substances that the human body either has no experience or not a good track record metabolizing.

Many people still don't realize that our bodies want to be healthy and are designed to stay healthy. However, we can't fool Mother Nature. We have to give our bodies the correct ingredients to properly do their jobs to keep us well.

If you're consuming a food or beverage created in a lab instead of by nature, you can be sure your body doesn't recognize it and know what to do with it. This opens the door to short-term and long-lasting health problems. When you expose your body to toxic influences, you deprive it of the nutritional building blocks it needs to stay healthy. Poor function, lack of vitality, and chronic disease then creep in over time.

The six Going Against GMOs for Optimal Health Eating Guidelines covered in this chapter all point to this: *Avoid the fake, heavily-tampered-with, chemical-laden, corporate-driven food impostors the food industry is pushing left and right on us, and eat organic, health-promoting, real food the body is designed for.* In our modern society, we all have become used to convenience foods and it's both a challenge and a process to keep avoiding GM foods and following the principles in this chapter. To do that, you definitely have to go against the status quo of what everyone else is eating. The more you can, the more you'll be giving your body the fuel it was designed for, and the healthier you will be.

Chapter 10 will provide information on how to shop non-GMO. Before that, though, the next chapter will give a rundown on various diets, from grain free to vegetarian to local, and explain where GM foods and other fake ingredients tend to hide and how to design each diet to promote optimal health.

Chapter 9:

Personalizing Going Against GMOs
for Specialty Diets

Some people are already following a specialty diet, such as a gluten-free diet, when they learn about GM foods and opt to also eliminate these untested food impostors. Others begin by avoiding GMOs, then they find they need a specialty diet, such as a gluten-free diet, for their best health. This chapter covers five popular styles of eating and how they fare in terms of avoiding the most common GM foods and following the nutrition guidelines for optimal health that were explained in the last chapter.

I specialize in gluten-free and grain-free omnivore diets. But in recent years I have counseled more people following vegetarian, vegan, organic, or local diets who sought my help to avoid GMOs or use other helpful nutrition strategies. I have become familiar with the problems people following a particular diet tend to encounter and where GMOs and other unnatural, unhealthy ingredients are apt to be. The purpose of this chapter is to share that information with you to help you fine-tune whatever diet you follow so it avoids the fake stuff that doesn't promote health and emphasizes real, whole foods.

GMOs and the chemical-based agriculture system we now have are issues that affect us all and will affect the future of our food and planet. They're too important for us to allow diet differences to get in the way. *No matter what type of diet we eat, it's time to honor our unique differences and work together to remove GMOs from our food supply and protect the integrity of our seeds, food system, and environment.* In an effort to help as many people as possible go non-GMO healthfully, the following is a summary on how to personalize going against GMOs for people following diets ranging from Paleolithic to vegan.

A GRAIN-FREE DIET

Though specifics may vary, grain-free diets cut out blood-sugar-spiking grain products often laden with GM ingredients, and avoid sugar, two important strategies for health. Some, however, emphasize meat and not many vegetables, while others allow artificial sweeteners or large amounts of dairy products, which derail health.

The most popular grain-free diet is *the Paleolithic diet* (also known as the hunter-gatherer or Stone Age diet), which is designed to approximate the types of foods our earliest ancestors ate. People who adopt a Paleolithic diet:

- Avoid all grain products including wheat, gluten, and corn
- Avoid all sweeteners (except, on occasion, small amounts of honey or maple syrup)
- Avoid all legumes, including soybeans
- Avoid all milk products
- Avoid all vegetable oils and partially hydrogenated oils
- Avoid all of the Big Five GM foods along with aspartame and rBGH in milk
- Eat whole foods instead of newfangled processed foods
- Eat a lot of non-starchy vegetables

Because *the Paleolithic diet adheres to pretty much all of the guidelines I covered in the last chapter and teaches people to eat whole foods and many vegetables,* I have found it extremely therapeutic for helping people lose weight and improving countless health conditions from autoimmune diseases to type 2 diabetes. The foundation of the Paleolithic diet is meat and non-starchy vegetables, along with high-quality fats, such as nuts and seeds, avocados, and olive oil or coconut oil, and smaller amounts of fruit. In my clinical experience, when people go from a standard American diet or even from a typical gluten-free diet to a Paleolithic diet, they improve so many nutritional aspects of their diet in one fell swoop (including avoiding all direct sources of GMOs), that they do very well on it, even when they eat commercial meat.

Nevertheless, until about 75 years ago, all animals used for meat were raised on organic pasture. Wild-caught fish, organic poultry, and grass-fed meat are less polluted and so much more nutritious than their conventional counterparts—and are from animals not fed GMOs—that I recommend that people gradually switch to wild-caught, organic, and grass-fed animal protein sources. Doing so is much better for health—both ours and the animals'—and it supports sustainable agriculture that works in concert with nature.

A Gluten-Free Diet

The gluten-free diet has become incredibly popular and even mainstream since I wrote *Going Against the Grain* in 2002. On a gluten-free diet:

- People strictly avoid gluten, found in wheat, rye, barley, and most oats, which is the only nutritional answer for solving gluten-related health problems in people with celiac disease or non-celiac gluten sensitivity.

- The rest of the diet can run the gamut from being based on naturally gluten-free whole foods to being more of a junk food gluten-free diet.

As a specialist in the gluten-free diet, I find that most gluten-free diet followers eat too many highly processed "gluten-free" products, such as bread, baked goods, and crackers. Doing this sets the stage for health problems in three different ways. The first way is, ironically, because those products are sometimes contaminated with unwanted gluten. Even though gluten-free grains and flours are naturally gluten free, these foods can inadvertently pick up gluten because they are often processed or stored in the same facilities as the gluten grains wheat, rye, and barley.

A study published in June 2010 by the *Journal of the American Dietetic Association* found that gluten contamination of inherently gluten-free grains and flours is common and should be a legitimate concern.

The second way gluten-free processed foods can lead to health problems is by prompting sharp increases in blood sugar and the fat-storage hormone insulin. Gluten-free foods made with ingredients such as rice flour, cornstarch, potato starch, and tapioca starch are high in carbohydrates and high on the glycemic index, meaning they are converted to sugar quickly and spike blood sugar levels. High blood sugar levels in turn set off a cascade of metabolic events that lead to uneven energy levels, increased hunger, addictive eating, unwanted weight gain, and a worsening of heart disease risk factors and prediabetic or diabetic blood sugar levels.

The third, lesser-known way that gluten-free convenience foods may contribute to health troubles is by being a source of genetically modified ingredients. Many gluten-free foods contain common GM ingredients such as: corn (i.e., cornstarch, cornmeal, corn syrup, corn oil, fructose, and xanthan gum); sugar from sugar beets (found in "sugar" listed in the list of ingredients or "beet sugar"); canola oil; and soy (i.e., soy flour, soy milk, tofu, soy oil, and soy lecithin). As you learned in Chapter 3, GM foods are linked to serious health risks, including reproductive problems, gastrointestinal problems, and immune system problems.

The healthiest way to eat gluten free is to emphasize naturally gluten-free foods, such as vegetables, fruits, meat, and nuts, but especially vegetables. When selecting packaged foods, seek out organic or Non-GMO Project Verified foods that are gluten-free certified, that have counter measures to avoid gluten contamination, or that test their ingredients, finished products, or equipment for gluten.

Also avoid any other food allergens you have and choose gluten-free whole grains such as wild rice or quinoa over refined rice flour or cornmeal products. In place of rice flour, potato starch, or cornmeal, try baking with almond flour (i.e., Dowd & Rogers or Honeyville) or coconut flour (i.e., Nutiva, Let's Do Organic, Bob's Red Mill, or Coconut Secret), which are lower glycemic, lower in carbohydrates, and richer in nutrients than traditional gluten-free flours.

A VEGETARIAN OR VEGAN DIET

Like gluten-free diets, there are many kinds of vegetarian (often called "plant-based" or "plant-strong") diets. Consider these key points:

- Vegans eat plant foods and avoid all animal products, including meat, fish, dairy products, and eggs.

- Vegetarians eat plant foods and include eggs and dairy products and sometimes fish on occasion.

- Either type of diet can be based on high-quality whole foods or can be based on low-quality processed vegetarian foods.

Vegetarians need to obtain adequate calories in their diet from some place other than meat—and they usually get their calories from grains, beans, eggs, dairy products, and fats. From working with vegetarians, I have been surprised how many of them eat too few vegetables and too many processed grain products that contain GMOs, refined flours, and refined vegetable oils. (These are frequent mistakes made by people on typical American or gluten-free diets, too.) It's also common for vegetarians to emphasize soy products, especially unfermented soy products, such as tofu, soy protein powder, and soy-based meat substitutes, which are usually GMO, and as I mentioned in the last chapter, are problematic in many other ways for health. Vegetarians not familiar with the GMO issue also eat many corn products, and some end up having sensitivities to foods they eat often, such as soy products or milk-based foods like cheese.

On a healthy vegetarian diet, as with other specialty diets, vegetables should be emphasized; blood-sugar-spiking sugar and flour/gluten-free flour products should be limited; and food allergens should be identified and avoided. If you choose to eat soy, corn, and milk products, select them carefully by looking for Non-GMO Project Verified and organic labels, and pay attention to how you feel when you eat these foods.

AN ORGANIC DIET

The numbers of people eating more organic foods have steadily increased in recent years. On an organic diet:

- People eat all or mostly organic foods, which means they automatically avoid GMOs, synthetic pesticides and fertilizers, sewage sludge and ionizing radiation, as well as antibiotics and growth hormones in meat.

- Some people may eat only organic whole foods, which is health promoting, while others may eat organic highly processed foods, such as organic sugar, white flour or gluten-free flour products, or vegetable oils, which contribute to disease, even though they are organic.

As a general rule, going organic is a great way to avoid GMOs and the other undesirable factors involved in industrial food production. The key to getting the most value out of organic foods, though, is emphasizing unprocessed whole foods and eating a lot of fresh produce. (As you probably have realized by now, this is a recurring theme in all therapeutic diets.)

I have found that some people are so focused on organic-only foods that they miss the fact that they'll get into health trouble regularly eating organic sugar and refined grains. They may start their day with an organic evaporated-cane-juice-sweetened cereal, eat organic bread, and treat themselves to organic cookies, even though they are overweight or have elevated blood sugar levels or other heart disease risk factors.

If you have a blood sugar- or insulin-related problem, you have to address it at its source, which are the many different forms of sugar in the diet. While organic sugar production is better for the environment and better for the body because it's free of synthetic pesticides, it makes no difference whether the sugar is from organic sugar or conventional sugar in terms of what it does to blood sugar and insulin levels and increasing the risk of many diseases, including cardiovascular disease and type 2 diabetes. I recommend going as organic as possible but I consider it equally important that you make sure to avoid disease-causing, refined food ingredients.

A LOCAL DIET

Emphasizing locally produced foods in the diet is a growing trend that's recommended by sustainable food experts. People who eat a local diet:

- Purchase all or mostly locally produced foods, especially locally grown fresh produce and locally produced meat, either at farmers' markets or directly from farms.

- Emphasize fresh foods at the peak of their season.

- Know that by purchasing local, they're making a big step toward reducing pollution and conserving our limited fuel sources, supporting local small businesses and farmers instead of large agrichemical corporations, and getting fresh food that is tastier and more nutritious than mass-market produced foods.

Eating more local foods is healthy and environmentally responsible in so many ways that it's a good dietary strategy for many people, especially if they have easy access to farmers' markets in their area. I especially like that buying local supports the agricultural system within the community, which all sustainable agriculture experts say is needed to improve the food system. Also, local food is fresher, so it tastes better.

The main downside of a local diet is that people assume that all foods sold at farmers' markets are free of pesticides or automatically good for them because they're local. Shoppers may ignore food sensitivities they have and may not ask enough questions, such as, "Do you grow these vegetables without pesticides?" or "Is your corn organic or heirloom?" They also tend to buy without looking at ingredients on sauces or packaged baked goods that clearly state sugar, cornstarch, canola oil, or soybean oil, which are of course undesirable. It's easy to correct those common mistakes by becoming a smart shopper. You'll learn the ins and outs of how to do that in the next chapter.

Putting It All Together

In this chapter I organized specialty diets into five general categories and made them sound black and white for the sake of simplicity. *The truth is there is a lot of overlapping going on among diets these days.* Many people who eat either a grain-free, omnivore diet or a vegan diet alternate between buying organic produce and buying local produce, depending on what's available. Some vegans also eat grain free because they don't tolerate grains well. Some Paleo diet eaters occasionally eat a vegan meal or a gluten-free grain like wild rice, while some vegans feel they need to eat wild-caught fish, organic chicken, or even an organic grass-fed burger on occasion.

There's a lot we can learn from the different diets outlined in this chapter, including the importance of avoiding harmful-to-health sugar, refined flours, and refined vegetable oils, and emphasizing health-promoting organic whole foods, particularly vegetables.

To make a specialty diet effective and therapeutic, it's essential to avoid making mistakes when you shop for food. The next chapter will teach you how to become a savvy non-GMO consumer, no matter where you shop.

Chapter 10:
How to Be a Savvy Non-GMO Shopper

Are you ready to build up your shopping knowledge to make healthy non-GMO food choices in the real world? This chapter will take you through the nuts and bolts of what to look for when shopping in conventional grocery stores, natural food supermarkets, and farmers' markets. In the next chapter, I'll share food ideas and recipes, and in Chapter 12, you'll learn all about eating out non-GMO.

Shopping savvy is covered first because purchasing high-quality, non-GMO foods is the most important factor for eating and cooking non-GMO at home. It's also covered first because the more you read food labels, the more you begin to understand the foods in which GMOs usually hide. You can then use that knowledge and transfer it to help you more easily eat non-GMO in restaurants.

GROCERY SHOPPING 101

As you likely have gathered by now, GMOs have infiltrated our food supply. That means unfortunately, there is not a lot of real food now sold in conventional supermarkets. More than 75 percent of the foods sold in grocery stores are estimated to contain genetically modified ingredients. About 80 percent of the 600,000 food items in America have added sugar, and other products contain additional harmful-to-health ingredients such as refined white flour, vegetable oils, trans-fats, and assorted food additives and preservatives you can't pronounce.

To seek out the real food, *avoid the inner aisles and shop mostly on the outer edges.* That is not only the best way to protect your health, it's also a simpler and much quicker way to shop.

You can select foods in the inner aisles of the grocery store but you have to be choosy about which ones you buy. Don't assume that a trusted iconic brand is automatically free from GMOs and don't be swayed by deceptive labeling and advertising.

It's exceptionally important to understand that "All Natural" on a product label doesn't mean the product is non-GMO. There is no formal definition for the use of "natural" on food labels that has been issued by the FDA or USDA. But "natural" is allowed on a food label of a product if the product does not contain added color, artificial flavors or synthetic substances and if the meat or poultry has had nothing added to the meat after slaughter. "Natural" certainly doesn't mean how the food was grown or raised. To make matters worse, the Grocery Manufacturers Association actually is trying to petition the U.S. Food and Drug Administration to allow foods that contain genetically modified ingredients to be able to be labeled "All Natural." If this were allowed to occur, it would be completely misleading because GM foods are anything but.

Although it's understandable to think that natural really means natural, do not be suckered into believing a product is *really* natural and free of GMOs if you see "All Natural" on a package. Instead of "All Natural," look instead for the Non-GMO Project Verified seal and the USDA Organic seal—or for unprocessed whole foods such as most vegetables that are not genetically modified

> Currently, all fresh vegetables and fruits sold in the United States are non-GMO except for three vegetables —yellow squash, zucchini, and sweet corn—and one fruit—papaya.

SHOPPING BASICS AT THE GROCERY STORE

The following is a quick guide of the ingredients to watch out for—and the foods you should emphasize—on a trip to the supermarket. GM ingredients are hidden in countless commercial products, so your best bet is to focus on fresh, unprocessed foods (those that have no label).

The Produce Section

One of the key guidelines for eating against GMOs for optimal health is to emphasize a wide variety of fresh vegetables and, to a lesser extent, fruits in your diet. That means you should spend much, if not most, of your time shopping in the produce department.

Fortunately, all vegetables and fruits in the produce department currently are non-GMO, except for three vegetables—yellow squash, zucchini, and sweet corn—and one fruit—papaya. Without adequate labeling, consumers can't know for sure which of these produce items are genetically modified, so it's best to seek out organic varieties of yellow squash, zucchini, and sweet corn (if you eat occasional corn on the cob).

Many stores do not even carry papaya. In the stores that do, completely avoid papaya grown in Hawaii or China and possibly look for Caribbean or Mexican red papayas, or avoid papaya altogether. (Some people wonder if we should avoid GM papaya because it's genetically modified to be virus resistant as opposed to being herbicide resistant like most GM crops. Keep in mind that genetically modifying any food can produce unpredictable changes in that food. GM papaya has never been proven safe and the Europe Union has enough concerns about it that the EU does not allow imports or cultivation of GM papaya.)

Non-starchy vegetables (in other words, non-root, non-winter squash, non-corn vegetables such as broccoli, asparagus, and spinach) should form the bulk of the produce you buy. That's especially true if you're sugar addicted or overweight. If you are not very sugar sensitive and don't need to lose weight, you can afford to experiment with virtually any fruit and vegetable, but watch how you feel after eating carbohydrate-dense vegetables and fruits, such as potatoes, tropical fruits and dried fruits. If you start to gain weight or have carbohydrate cravings from eating these foods, that's a clear sign you need to reduce your intake or avoid them and stick solely to non-starchy vegetables.

THE LOWDOWN ON PRODUCE

Fruits and vegetables are better in countless ways for health than even organic refined grain-based foods, so fruits and vegetables should be emphasized in the diet, even if they are conventionally grown.

To avoid GMOs, buy organic zucchini and yellow squash—or buy Mexican grey squash or heirloom summer squash instead—and avoid commercial corn on the cob and papaya unless you're assured they're non-GMO.

Then go further in upgrading the quality of the produce you eat. If you can't afford to always buy organic, **reduce exposure to pesticides by choosing organic varieties of the worst pesticide-laden produce items listed below**. They include the Environmental Working Group's (EWG's) so-called Dirty Dozen (from 2014), which have high concentrations of pesticides on them, plus a few extra vegetables, kale, collard greens, and hot peppers, which are frequently contaminated with insecticides that are toxic to the human nervous system, according to the EWG.

The Best Produce Items to Buy Organic*

Apple	Potatoes
Celery	Snap peas (imported)
Cherry Tomatoes	Spinach
Cucumbers	Strawberries
Grapes	Sweet and hot peppers
Nectarines (imported)	Kale and collard greens
Peaches	

*Includes the Dirty Dozen + the Dirty Dozen Plus list for 2014 as assessed by the Environmental Working Group

Beyond avoiding both genetically modified and carbohydrate-dense vegetables and fruits, my consistent advice is to buy organic varieties of produce—those grown without synthetic pesticides—whenever possible. If you can't always buy organic, at least try to choose organic varieties of the most pesticide-laden produce items. Some 65 percent of thousands of produce samples analyzed by the U.S. Department of Agriculture test positive for pesticide residues, and European regulators have banned several pesticides the United States uses, yet the Environmental Protection Agency (EPA) has not complied with a law passed in 1996 to tell Americans ways they can reduce pesticides in their diets.

To remedy that problem, every year for more than a decade, the non-profit Environmental Working Group has stepped in where the EPA has not by publishing a Shopper's Guide to Pesticides in Produce. The guide, which you can learn more about at EWG.org, lists the most pesticide-contaminated conventional produce, what EWG calls the "Dirty Dozen."

Organics unfortunately are not easily accessible or affordable for everyone, so paying attention to the list can help people who watch their money choose organic on the riskiest produce items. The list changes every year according to updated data, so visit EWG.org for the most recent list.

However, certain items, such as apples, strawberries, peaches, imported nectarines, sweet bell peppers, and spinach are regularly on the Dirty Dozen list. Avocados, onions, asparagus, sweet potatoes, and kiwi usually tend to have the least amount of pesticide residues.

The Meat and Seafood Sections

In the meat and seafood sections of the store, keep in mind that all fresh meat and seafood is not genetically engineered. (If GM salmon is allowed on the market, this would be an exception to the rule. However, if GM salmon is allowed on the market, many supermarkets have pledged not to sell it.) Though not direct sources of GMOs, conventional animal protein sources are from animals fed GM feed, meaning they're indirect sources. Avoiding indirect sources of GMOs is step 2 of taking GMOs out of our diets and out of the food supply.

When you're beginning to remove GMOs out of your diet—or if you eat a typical American diet or a grain-free Paleolithic diet—choosing conventional meat items in traditional supermarkets is often necessary to keep blood sugar levels steady and avoid eating even more unhealthy GMO-laden, refined sugar- and flour-based products, which make up most of the items in the store. When you are able to, seek out organic poultry and organic grass-fed meats as much as you can from natural food supermarkets and farmers' markets.

If you can't because of a lack of finances or lack of access to these options, I recommend that you avoid commercial beef entirely and choose lamb instead. Lamb is not eaten in the amount that beef is in the United States and therefore lambs are not raised in the GMO-laden feed lots that cattle are. American lamb may still be given some grain but not in the amounts and conditions that cattle are fed. If you find lamb from Australia, there's a better chance it's 100 percent grass fed, and if you find lamb from New Zealand, that's even better.

To avoid hidden sources of GMOs and other risky-to-health food additives in animal protein sources, choose unprocessed meats or poultry. Avoid meats and poultry that are prebasted, deep basted, premarinated, breaded, smoked and cured, or made into sausage.

In the seafood department, avoid farm-raised fish, which are typically fed GM pellets. Look for wild-caught fish instead.

The Refrigerator Sections

If you aren't allergic to eggs, which are a common food allergen, seek out organic eggs, which many conventional grocery stores now carry. Organic eggs are from chickens fed organic feed, usually organic corn and soy.

As I explained in Chapter 8, most of my clients experience their best health eating no milk products at all. However, if you eat some milk products such as butter or cheese without experiencing uncomfortable symptoms, be sure to look for organic dairy products. Many traditional grocery stores don't offer organic milk products, so you might have to go to natural food stores to find them.

To clarify, milk used for organic dairy items are from cows that are fed organic feed and are not treated with antibiotics or genetically modified recombinant bovine growth hormone (rBGH). Cows treated with rBGH have higher levels of insulin growth factor 1 (IGF-1), and consuming high levels of IGF-1 is associated with higher levels of cancer.

The Frozen Foods Section

In the frozen foods section of the supermarket, bypass all the heavily processed frozen meals and party foods, and stick with frozen vegetables and frozen fruit. Frozen vegetables last a lot longer than fresh vegetables and are ready to cook at a moment's notice. It's a good idea to buy several different types of frozen vegetables and have them in your freezer to help you "veg" out and continue to eat against GMOs at times when you're out of fresh vegetables or just too busy or tired to chop them.

Always read the list of ingredients on packages in the frozen food section carefully and make sure these products contain no additives or hidden ingredients. Avoid Dirty Dozen vegetables and fruits, unless they are organic, when possible, and avoid corn and edamame, which are young soybeans.

Quick Stops in the Inner Aisles

The inner aisles of a traditional supermarket aren't places to spend much time in because GMOs, sugar, and refined not-good-for-you ingredients abound in most of the products. The following are some of the healthiest choices you might want on your shopping list as well as a few important reminders of what to avoid.

Beans and Grains

Most of my clients avoid beans and grains entirely and feel better doing so. However, if you eat a vegetarian/vegan diet, or if you can tolerate higher amounts of carbohydrates without experiencing carbohydrate cravings, gaining weight, or feeling digestive distress, the good news is that all beans except for soybeans are non-GMO.

The bad news is that canned beans often contain GM oils and other hidden GM ingredients and food additives. Look for bags of unprocessed dry beans, preferably organic dry beans that you cook yourself—or cans of organic beans, such as those by Amy's Organic Kitchen.

The three best tolerated grains or grain-like alternatives are gluten-free wild rice, quinoa, and brown rice. It's often difficult to find wild rice in conventional supermarkets, but occasionally you can, and quinoa, such as Ancient Harvest quinoa, is often available.

Brown rice deserves a special explanation. It's not well known, but in 2006 an unapproved GM rice variety known as Liberty Link 601 somehow escaped from field trials in the southern United States and contaminated some U.S. rice stocks. The contamination greatly hurt some companies' U.S. rice exports to other countries and caused companies such as Lundberg Family Farms to test their products and replace some rice ingredients with California-grown rice products.[142] [143] For this reason, I recommend seeking out Non-GMO Project Verified and USDA Organic rice products, such as Lundberg Family Farms, which you fortunately can usually find in conventional supermarkets.

Nuts

Nutrient-dense nuts make convenient snack foods and tasty salad and entree toppers, and research shows that eating nuts regularly in the diet confers many health benefits, including reducing the risk of type 2 diabetes, cardiovascular disease, sudden cardiac death, and macular degeneration. Contrary to what most people believe, people actually lose weight better on nut-rich diets, and those who eat nuts are leaner than those who don't.[144] I consider them a very good addition to most people's diets, unless of course people are allergic to them.

The key is to avoid nuts roasted in GM vegetable oils, such as canola oil, soybean oil, corn oil, or cottonseed oil. Purchase raw or dry roasted nuts instead. Look for raw nuts without additives such as BHA and BHT in the baking aisle of your local supermarket. You also can sometimes find raw nuts, such as pecan or walnut halves or sliced almonds, in stands in the store's produce section.

To find dry roasted nuts, look in the snack food aisle of the store. Select those that say they are dry roasted and do not contain any other ingredients other than nuts. Blue Diamond is a brand that you can find in most stores. Avoid Blue Diamond's flavored varieties of almonds, and select its whole natural almonds or unsalted dry roasted almonds.

Canned Foods, Condiments, & Seasonings

Commercial canned foods and condiments almost always contain vegetable oils, sugar, distilled white vinegar or citric acid, which are usually derived from GM corn, and many other undesirable food additives. It's best to look for "clean," organic versions of these items, such as sun-dried tomatoes in olive oil, artichoke hearts, or even salsa, in health food stores.

Also beware that all commercial salad dressings should be avoided. Salad dressings sound healthy, but they're made with vegetable oils, typically from GM sources, xanthan gum, which is usually derived from

GM corn, and other harmful-to-health food additives, including sugar. It's best to make your own dressing at home with a good-quality extra virgin olive oil and an organic red wine vinegar or a balsamic vinegar with no sugar added, or with olive oil, lemon juice and herbs.

In the ethnic or Asian foods aisle of the store, there's a canned food that's a boon to most people who go against GMOs and dairy products: Canned lite or regular unsweetened coconut milk. Thai Kitchen is one brand to look for. Try it in place of milk or cream in coffee or tea, on top of fresh pineapple cubes or thawed frozen cherries, or in place of highly processed, sugar-laden milk alternatives such as soy milk and rice milk in recipes and baking.

Beverages

Cutting sugar out of the beverages you drink is one of the most important ways to dramatically improve your health. Steer clear not only of fruit drinks, soft drinks, and tea and coffee beverages sweetened with GM high-fructose corn syrup and sugar, but also fruit juices. Even though they're more natural than soft drinks, fruit juices are liquid sugars that are concentrated sources of fructose, which set people up for weight gain and conditions such as high blood triglycerides.

Water, the only beverage that is a nutrient all by itself, should be your go-to drink. Buy bottled water, sparkling mineral water or sparkling water with flavor essences at the grocery store—or consider purchasing a high-quality, reverse-osmosis water filter for your home. For a non-dairy source of calcium, look for a high-calcium sparkling mineral water, such as San Pellegrino.

Organic and Non-GMO Project Verified Foods

Many grocery stores now carry some foods labeled USDA Organic. With some major food companies such as Post Cereals announcing that its Grape-Nuts cereal is now Non-GMO Project Verified, you should expect to see more products sold in traditional supermarkets carry the Non-GMO Project seal in the coming months and years.

The process in the food industry generally goes like this: Natural food stores set trends by offering food options that health-conscious customers want. When a food trend becomes more popular than what is considered a "niche" market, conventional supermarkets follow. That happened with gluten free, it happened with organic, and now that process has begun with Non-GMO Project Verified.

Some traditional grocery stores have so-called "health foods" in a special section of the store. In other stores, Non-GMO Project Verified and organic products are interspersed among conventional products.

In either case, to be the most informed non-GMO shopper you can be and make the best purchasing decisions possible, it's important to understand exactly what the Non-GMO Project Verified label and the USDA Organic label really mean. Far too many people think the two labels mean the same thing.

In the next few pages, you'll learn the details of how each label differs and the benefits and drawbacks of each one. In a nutshell, Non-GMO Project Verified means the product has passed a process-based program that involves traceability, segregation and testing at critical control points to verify that products are not genetically modified. USDA Organic goes beyond just avoiding GMOs by avoiding many other undesirable outputs used in conventional agriculture.

NON-GMO VS. ORGANIC:
Understanding the Difference

Both are good ways to avoid GMOs yet they have definable distinctions.

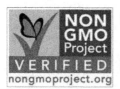 Non-GMO Project Verified

In order to earn the Non-GMO Project Verified label, a product must undergo a rigorous review process by the non-profit organization, the Non-GMO Project, which operates North America's only third party verification program for GMO avoidance. The verification program includes testing of at-risk ingredients on an ongoing basis. The ingredients that are tested—crops currently in production in genetically engineered form—include alfalfa, canola, corn, cotton, papaya, soy, sugar beets, yellow squash, and zucchini. Animal products, including milk, meat, eggs, and honey, are also tested.[145]

The only focus of the program is GMO avoidance. A product could meet the standards of GMO avoidance but still could contain ingredients that are grown with commercial pesticides, which many health-conscious shoppers also want to avoid.

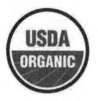 USDA Organic

The use of GMOs is prohibited under the United States Department of Agriculture (USDA) National Organic Program. To meet the USDA organic regulations, farmers and processors must show they aren't using GMOs and also that they are protecting their products from contact with GMOs through a variety of methods, such as implementing "buffer zones" next to GMO fields, delaying planting or doing early planting to avoid organic and GMO crops flowering at the same time, and using properly cleaned farm equipment.[146] That's why the USDA Organic seal on products automatically means non-GMO to most people.

However, organic certification does not require testing for GMOs. Given the widespread use of GMOs, and some GM crops such as corn being notorious for spreading through wind drift and contaminating other fields, some shoppers want the extra insurance of GMO testing and opt for the Non-GMO Project Verified label for that reason.

There are many more reasons to buy USDA Organic food than just to avoid GMOs. A driving factor for many people is they want to support a beneficial food production system that sustains the health of soils, the environment, and people.[147] Another big factor is the desire to avoid health-disruptive substances that are excluded from organic farming—not just GMOs, but also irradiation, sewage sludge, antibiotics, growth hormones, and synthetic chemical fertilizers and pesticides, many of which have been linked to a number of health problems, including neurologic and endocrine (hormone) system disorders and cancer.[148] [149] When shoppers purchase organic, they know they not only reduce their exposure to pesticides, but also spare farm workers who work in the fields from that pesticide exposure.

Still another good reason to purchase organic foods is because they're more nutritious. Reviews of multiple studies show that organic foods provide significantly greater levels of vitamin C, iron, magnesium and phosphorus than non-organic varieties of the same foods. They also tend to provide greater levels of health-supporting antioxidant phytochemicals, such as flavonoids,[150] and a 2013 study found that organically produced milk has a more beneficial fatty acid composition helpful for promoting reduced inflammation in the body.[151]

MAKING AN EDUCATED CHOICE

Non-GMO Verified products generally cost less than certified organic foods, so if you can't always afford organic foods but want to avoid GMOs, buy non-GMO, especially for products that contain the main ingredients at risk to contain GMOs.

If you want to avoid GMOs but also think there are too many pesticides and other undesirable practices in conventional agriculture and want to use your purchasing power to buy food that's produced in ecologically protective ways, buy organic.

You actually don't have to choose just one of these labels. You can choose both. More than half of the Non-GMO Project's verified products are certified organic. If you want the extra protection of both programs for GMO avoidance together, if you want the food that you purchase to have been tested for GMOs, and if you also want to use your dollars to support the many benefits of organic agriculture, choose products with both the Non-GMO Project Verified label and USDA Organic label. The two seals together are the gold standard at the present time for signifying unadulterated pure food as nature intended.

HOW NATURAL FOOD STORES ARE DIFFERENT

Although there are relatively slim pickings of non-GMO food products available in conventional grocery stores, there are many more options for eating non-GMO and organic in natural food stores. To more easily eat non-GMO, I recommend shopping in natural food supermarkets, especially in ones that offer fresh meats and produce, and also at farmers' markets.

With that said, it's important not to be overwhelmed by all the options and make poor purchasing decisions. Poor decisions made in natural food stores or specialty food stores can derail your health just like poor decisions made elsewhere. Never assume that everything sold in natural food stores is free of GMOs or that everything there is healthy for you, no matter how healthy the words on labels sound. Instead, be a discriminating shopper by reading labels carefully, following the guidelines for eating non-GMO covered in Chapter 6 and for eating for optimal health covered in Chapter 8, and understanding the difference between non-GMO and organic.

To make informed decisions about what to buy, know the different ways natural food stores offer healthier alternatives to the products found in grocery stores. First, natural food supermarkets carry a wider selection of organic products—foods not sprayed with pesticides—and sometimes organic locally grown produce, such as what you might find at farmers' markets. Most natural food supermarkets also offer: many clearly-labeled USDA Organic and Non-GMO Project Verified products, including meats; meats, eggs and dairy products from animals not treated with added growth hormones or antibiotics; many gluten-free and grain-free food products; and "cleaner" convenience foods with much fewer additives.

Beware that not all natural food and specialty food stores are the same. Different stores have different policies. Let me explain the examples of Trader Joe's and Whole Foods Market. Trader Joe's says their private label products contain no genetically engineered ingredients. However, no independent third-party certifier verifies that their products are non-GMO on a regular basis. The chain shrouds its non-GMO claims in secrecy and won't share names of companies that produce the products and won't share affidavits that show any proof of non-GMO corn or soy in non-organic products. Without any verification, I can't trust that Trader Joe's products are truly non-GMO. Neither can Vani Hari, known as Food Babe, who after investigating the matter wrote an article on her Foodbabe.com site entitled, "What Is Trader Joe's Hiding?" Whole Foods, by contrast, already offers a large selection of clearly labeled independently tested Non-GMO Project Verified products and will require labeling of all foods sold in their stores that aren't organic or Non-GMO Project Verified by 2018.

Trader Joe's still sells some meat from animals raised on antibiotics, while Whole Foods Market does not allow antibiotics in any of the meats it sells.[152] Consumers Union has launched a campaign against Trader Joe's to stop this practice because the overuse of antibiotics on healthy animals by meat and poultry industries is promoting the spread of drug-resistant superbugs that threaten public health.

In addition, Whole Foods has a list of more than 75 ingredients it does not consider acceptable for foods sold in its stores—numerous unhealthy ingredients I mentioned in Chapter 8, such as: partially hydrogenated oil; high-fructose corn syrup; irradiated foods; monosodium glutamate; the artificial sweeteners aspartame, saccharin, and sucralose; artificial colors; artificial flavors; and numerous food additives like nitrites/nitrates and BHA and BHT.[153] There are some other ingredients and additives it would be good for Whole Foods to add to its list, but its unacceptable ingredients list is way better than most chains. Earth Fare, a chain of natural food supermarkets in North Carolina, the southeastern United States, and Ohio, has a "Boot list" of ingredients it has banned from its shelves that includes high-fructose corn syrup, artificial fats or artificial trans fats, artificial colors, artificial flavors, artificial preservatives, artificial sweeteners, antibiotics or synthetic growth hormones in fresh meat or dairy, and bleached or bromated flour. Trader Joe's, on the other hand, doesn't appear to have a list of ingredients that it won't accept.

Many people have somehow acquired the idea that everything sold at Trader Joe's is non-GMO or organic and "safe." That definitely is not true, and I wanted to fill you in on the details so you know what a misconception that is. Don't get me wrong: You still can buy healthy non-GMO foods at Trader Joe's. I shop there as well as many other places, including Whole Foods, locally owned natural food stores, and farmers' markets. However, to be a savvy shopper, it's important to avoid jumping to unrealistic conclusions about your favorite stores and be more discerning when you shop.

GOING THE EXTRA MILE: SHOPPING IN NATURAL FOOD STORES

I find that that there's consumer-oriented information that most people don't know but want and need to know when they shop in natural food stores. To keep shopping easy for you, I've compiled that information so you can make savvy choices to best support your health when you shop in health food stores.

The Produce Section

Even in a natural food store, the cautions I've already mentioned about avoiding GM produce items (yellow squash, zucchini, corn on the cob, and papaya) and the Dirty Dozen (including popular fruits such as apples and strawberries), unless they are organic, still apply. If you see something like fresh papaya or corn on the cob in a natural food store, don't assume it's non-GMO just because it's sold in a health food store. The chances are good that it is genetically modified.

If you don't know, ask the produce manager. If he gives you an answer that you wonder about or don't know whether to trust, skip buying it. Just politely let the produce manager know that buying non-GMO is an important issue to you. If you do the simple act of talking to the produce manager and asking about whether the produce item is non-GMO, the natural food store will understand that growing numbers of people want Non-GMO Project Verified versions of the at-risk fruits and vegetables that customers can count on.

Sometimes I get questions about potatoes and tomatoes. Here's the scoop: Although genetically engineered potatoes and tomatoes were developed and briefly introduced long ago, both products failed in marketplace. For quite some time now, there have been no genetically modified potatoes and tomatoes in commercial production. Both are usually heavily sprayed with pesticides, though, so it's a good idea to buy organic varieties of these items.

I've sometimes heard clients complain about how expensive produce sold in natural food supermarkets is. As I've mentioned throughout this book, fresh vegetables and smaller amounts of fruits are the most health-promoting types of carbohydrates to spend your money on, and it's important to eat a wide variety of vegetables, such as asparagus, Globe artichokes, broccoli, cabbage, kale, and spinach. It's far better to spend more money on produce than on a bunch of packaged Non-GMO Project Verified products.

Also, many natural food stores carry organic produce and some carry locally grown produce. As I previously explained, organic farmers and small local farmers who grow fruits and vegetables don't get the subsidies that large corporate food companies do. Many of my clients understand that it's better to pay more upfront on food and stay well in the long term than to buy many cheap food products and pay more in health care later. It's also better to vote with your dollars and support farmers who are growing food the way it should be grown. When you consider the big picture, buying organic helps farm workers and helps the environment. Buying locally grown foods helps keep more money in your community, generally tastes fresher and better, and saves energy because there is much less transportation from farm to store.

All that said, I completely understand when finances are an issue. Can you imagine getting a pint of organic blueberries for 99 cents, or a pound of organic 100% grass-fed ground beef for $3.99? You can get those deals and many others if you simply pay attention to the weekly ads of natural food stores in your area, or sign up for email bulletins of special sales they do. When you carefully monitor ads and special sales from your favorite stores, you can compare prices on the items you most want, and be able to buy organic produce (and other food items) for the same price or less than conventional produce and products.

The Fish, Poultry, and Meat Departments

Everything sold in the meat case of natural food stores is not non-GMO. The following labeling terms—All Natural, Cage Free, Free Range, Certified Humanely Raised, Vegetarian Diet, Fair Trade, and Locally Grown—have no direct relevance to whether a product is GMO free. *To avoid animal protein sources from animals fed GM feed, look for organic and Non-GMO Project Verified meats and poultry, and wild-caught fish.* Examples of wild-caught fish include wild sockeye salmon, wild Alaskan halibut, and wild-caught mahi-mahi.

In the poultry section, you have to sort through many options. You'll often find conventional chicken (from chickens fed GM feed), as well as Non-GMO Project Verified chicken and USDA Organic chicken. The difference between the latter two is that Non-GMO Verified chicken receives Non-GMO Project Verified feed, but is not raised according to organic standards. Organic chicken means the chicken must be fed organic feed without GMOs and without persistent pesticides and chemical fertilizers for its entire life. The bird must have outdoor access and cannot be given drugs, antibiotics, or growth hormones. Organic chicken costs a little more than Non-GMO Project Verified, but it's better in terms of avoiding problematic chemicals and drugs. If you can't buy organic chicken, Non-GMO Project Verified chicken is a good option. Mary's Chicken now offers both Non-GMO Project Verified chicken and USDA Organic chicken. For those on a tight budget, an especially good buy is organic chicken livers, which you can usually purchase for less than a dollar per serving.

There's another very important issue for health: getting meat as much as possible from animals raised on grass, or open pasture, instead of non-GMO corn and soy. Chickens and pigs raised on pasture require some higher-protein supplemental feed from foods such as corn and soy. But ruminant animals such as cattle and bison are meant to eat grass alone. They have trouble digesting large amounts of grain because they lack a critical enzyme needed to metabolize starch. These animals have to be slowly introduced to an unnatural diet of corn and soy. Even after adapting to it, they often are sick with conditions such as acidosis and liver abscesses, and they're treated with antibiotics and medications.

The way to solve this problem is to get back to meat as close to the way it was 100 years ago: organic and pasture raised. It's better for the health of the animals, better for us, and better for the environment.

Compared with feedlot meat, meat from grass-fed beef, bison, lamb and goats is much more nutritious. Consider these benefits:

- Grass-fed meat has less total fat, saturated fat, cholesterol, and calories. (Get this: grass-fed beef can have the same amount of fat as skinless chicken breast, wild deer, or elk!)

- It has more vitamin E, beta-carotene, vitamin C, and a number of health-promoting fats, including anti-inflammatory omega-3 fatty acids and conjugated linoleic acid, or CLA, which has fat-burning properties and may be a potent cancer fighter.[154] [155]

- It carries a lower risk of harmful *E. coli* and *campylobacter* bacteria, studies suggest. [156] [157] [158]

There's another benefit: Not using grain in meat production helps the environment in numerous ways, says author Jo Robinson in *Why Grassfed is Best.* It eliminates the herbicides and fertilizers used to grow large amounts of corn that are fed to cattle, and eliminates the oil and natural gas used in mowers and combines to harvest the grain and in vehicles to ship the grain to the animals or the animals to the grain.[159]

Grass fed, pastured, and pasture raised are terms that are not regulated or certified, so keep in mind two important points when shopping. *First, organic meat is not the same as pasture-raised meat.* Animals raised organically are not given hormones or antibiotics to promote growth, and they eat only organic feed, such as organic corn and soy, without any pesticides or animal by-products. But that does not mean they are raised on organic pasture unless the meat is labeled both certified organic and grass fed.

Second, all animals are raised on pasture for some or most of their lives but most animals are "finished" or fattened up on grain. To avoid GMOs and to get all of the benefits attributed to grass-fed meat, look for meat that is both *grass fed and grass finished,* or labeled *100% grass fed,* as well as *organic.* Sommers, Eel River, and Panorama organic grass-fed meats are three such brands. Mindful Meats, the first Non-GMO Project Verified beef company in the United States, is another. New Zealand lamb, is 100% grass fed and not given antibiotics.

You can also search for local organic grass-fed meat, poultry, egg, and dairy companies in your area at Eatwild.com, which lists a directory of pasture-based farms across the country. You usually can only find organic, pasture-raised chicken at farmers' markets or directly from farms. Standards vary, so be sure to double-check with local meat companies to make certain they do not feed their animals conventional alfalfa, corn, soy, or other typical GM ingredients.

Also, keep in mind that different brands of 100 percent grass-fed meat may vary in taste. If you don't like one brand, try another.

The Refrigerator Sections

In the refrigerated sections of natural food stores, you can usually find Non-GMO Project Verified eggs from chickens that have been fed non-GMO feed. Brands of Non-GMO Project Verified eggs include Nature Fed and NestFresh.

If you can afford to invest a bit more in your health, buy organic eggs, which are from chickens fed organic feed. Even better for your health are organic, pasture-raised eggs. Vital Farms is one brand of organic, pasture-raised eggs that's easy to find in Whole Foods Markets nationwide. Vital Farms also offers pasture-raised, Non-GMO Project Verified eggs named Backyard Eggs, which aren't as widely available.

As I previously mentioned, most people do best eating no or very few milk products. If you eat some milk products, such as butter or cheese, keep in mind the same steps for going non-GMO and beyond as I discussed with meat and eggs:

Non-GMO Project Verified—from cows fed non-GM feed

↓

USDA Organic—from cows fed organic feed and raised according to organic standards (not given antibiotics or hormones)

↓

Organic, Pasture-Raised—from cows raised according to organic standards and raised on organic pasture

Just like pasture-raised meats and poultry, pasture-raised dairy products contain more beneficial omega-3 fatty acids and more beta-carotene, and the production of them is better for the environment. Organic Valley makes both organic butter and organic, pasture butter. The Rumiano Cheese Company's entire line of organic cheeses is Non-GMO Project Verified and made from milk from grass-fed cows.

In April 2014, the natural foods chain Natural Grocers by Vitamin Cottage made a major announcement that its nearly 90 stores will no longer sell dairy products that come from confinement dairies. (In a confinement dairy, the animals do not graze on growing pasture and live their unnaturally shortened lives enclosed in a barn or dirt yard.) Instead, Natural Grocers will only sell dairy products from animals that are pasture raised. The process of ensuring that all products are pasture-based and phasing out products from confinement dairies will take about a year.

Quick Stops in the Inner Aisles

It's relatively easy now to find Non-GMO Project Verified or USDA organic foods and beverages of about every type imaginable in natural food stores. Please keep in mind, though, that many of the foods with these labels are packaged foods with refined ingredients that we should be avoiding or limiting in our diet. Remember that choosing conventional non-GMO fresh vegetables that don't have any labels is better for health than choosing highly refined grain products that contain refined vegetable oils and have Non-GMO Project Verified or organic labels on them.

Unlike other non-GMO shopping guides, I won't be listing non-GMO foods high in sugar and other not-good-for-you refined ingredients. Though I understand that people may occasionally buy foods that aren't perfect as "treats" or social party foods, the information about types of foods and specific products that I provide below is advice I give my clients to steer them to real food that supports health day in and day out over the long term. It is based on my personal experience as an independent nutritionist and is meant to be used as a healthy non-GMO products guide.

The Frozen Foods Section

Read the list of ingredients on packages in the frozen food section carefully and make sure these products contain no additives or hidden ingredients. I recommend avoiding cut corn and edamame (a soy product) altogether. Also avoid Dirty Dozen vegetables and fruits, unless they are organic, when possible.

Keep an eye out for organic fruits and vegetables on sale, and stock up on them when they're at a good price so you have them ready to use when you run out of fresh produce. Most frozen meals and snacks tend to be too processed or too high in carbohydrates, and often contain GMOs and/or vegetable oils or sugar.

However, for vegetarians or meat eaters who can handle higher amounts of carbs without adverse health effects, the following are two organic frozen foods that are made with real food that can make for fast food or convenient side dishes:

WHAT TO LOOK FOR
WHEN SHOPPING FOR MEAT AND POULTRY

Less than a century ago, the poultry and meat that Americans ate were from animals naturally raised on organic pasture. Today most commercially available meat is from animals fed an unnatural diet of herbicide-sprayed, genetically engineered corn and soy.

To avoid meat from animals fed GM feed, look for any of the following labels. To purchase the highest quality poultry and meat that is more in keeping with the non-industrially produced types eaten by our ancestors, choose organic and pasture-raised or 100% grass-fed whenever possible.

Poultry:

Organic, Pasture-Raised Poultry (raised on organic pasture including insects, or on organic pasture and organic grains and legumes)

Organic Poultry (fed organic feed, typically organic corn & soy)

Non-GMO Project Verified Poultry (fed non-GM feed, typically non-GM corn and soy)

Meat:

Organic 100% Grass-fed (grass-fed and grass-finished) Meats

Non-GMO Project Verified, Pasture-Raised Meats

100% Grass-Fed Lamb from New Zealand

Organic Meats (typically fed organic corn and soy)

Non-GMO Project Verified Meats (fed non-GM corn and soy)

- *Asherah's Gourmet 100% organic vegan burgers.* These unique, all-organic burgers are made with the South American gluten-free super-"grain" quinoa (which isn't really a grain), sweet potato, carrots, other vegetables, and flaxseeds. Available in

original and chipotle flavor, the easy-to-fix burgers are free of
the top ten food allergens and packed with vitamin A, B-6, iron,
magnesium, and fiber.

- *Organic Sunshine Burgers.* These convenient soy-free vegan
  burgers are made with organic cooked brown rice, organic ground
  sunflower seeds and other organic ingredients. They're available
  in seven different flavors, including Garden Herb, Mushroom,
  and Falafel.

Beans and Gluten-Free Grains

Some additional advice for vegetarians or those on higher-carbohydrate
diets: Beans such as garbanzo beans, kidney beans, and pinto beans,
generally keep blood sugar levels steadier than grains. Look for bags
of dry beans or canned beans from Eden Organic, Westbrae Organic, or
organic varieties from Whole Foods' 365 brand. Among canned beans,
Eden tends to have the cleanest ingredients.

When grains are eaten, naturally gluten-free quinoa, wild rice, and
brown rice are the ones that tend to be best tolerated. Neither quinoa nor
wild rice is a member of the grain family. Quinoa has all the amino acids
needed to make a complete protein and is easy for most people to digest.

Wild rice is lower in carbohydrates and calories than brown rice and
other grains—it has 25 fewer calories and 5 fewer grams of carbohydrate
than brown rice per half-cup serving—so some people who are sensitive
to grains or carbohydrates tolerate wild rice well.

Rice is the best tolerated member of the grain family. Earlier in this
chapter, I explained why it's important to seek out a Non-GMO Project
Verified, organic variety of rice, such as Lundberg Farms.

Another Non-GMO Project Verified, USDA Organic brand of rice that's
important to know about is Lotus Foods. This company sells three
types of rice produced through a set of ecologically sound concepts

and practices known as the System of Rice Intensification (SRI) that has changed the way rice is typically grown. Developed in Madagascar in the early 1980s, SRI methods enable farmers with limited resources to increase their rice yields using 80 to 90 percent less seed, 25 to 50 percent less water, and few or no chemical fertilizers and pesticides. The farmers are able to use seeds of the traditional varieties of rice they have historically grown. To help protect resources and the environment, consider purchasing a SRI rice. Types of SRI-grown rice available from Lotus Foods include: Organic Madagascar Pink Rice, Organic Brown Jasmine Rice, Organic Brown Mekong Flower Rice, and Organic Volcano Rice. As an added bonus for consumers, they cook in less time than brown rice.

Though I find many people do best not eating corn processed into shells and tortillas because of their high-glycemic effects, if you occasionally splurge on some Mexican food, the 365 brand of Organic Blue Corn Taco Shells, which are Non-GMO Project Verified in addition to being organic, are one of the best choices available. The taco shells are particularly fun for kids who like to make their own tacos.

Nuts, Seeds, and Nut Butters

Nuts, seeds, and nut butters all come in handy to use as snacks. However, bags of organic nuts are hard to come across. When they are available, products such as Essential Living Foods organic almonds and cashews, and Living Intentions' Gone Nuts raw and sprouted nut blends, are out of the price range most of my clients can afford.

If you can't find or afford organic nuts, Trader Joe's is a convenient place to buy nuts that are not organic. The chain offers a wide variety, such as slivered toasted almonds or raw or dry roasted almonds, all for a good price.

Organic sprouted seeds, such as sunflower or pumpkin seeds, are a little more affordable. Hail Merry offers sprouted organic sunflower seeds, and Go Raw offers sprouted sunflower and sprouted pumpkin seeds.

Nut butter makes a great addition to many people's (especially vegans') diets. Nut butter on celery sticks or apple slices are blood-sugar-stabilizing snacks. Raw organic nut butters, such as those from Artisana, are delicious, but they too tend to be too expensive to buy regularly. One product that is worth the extra cost to many of my clients, especially those who follow a grain-free Paleolithic diet, is Nutiva Coconut Manna. Just a tablespoon of it makes a satisfying low-carb treat.

Though many nut butters are available, almond butter is the nut butter most of my clients do best eating because it has a more even balance of protein and carbohydrates. For a good buy, purchase unsalted, unsweetened, roasted almond butter at Trader Joe's or the 365 brand at Whole Foods.

Snack Foods

The best snack foods are ones made from nutrient-dense, grain-free, whole foods, such as flavorful vegetables, herbs, and sometimes nuts and seeds. They take snacking to a whole new level. Sure, the following may seem expensive. However, because they are made of nutrient-dense whole foods, they satisfy you in a way that high-glycemic corn or potato chips don't. You'll find you don't need many to take the edge off hunger. In addition to being super-nutritious organic snack foods, they also make great toppers to salads when they're crumbled. As with all health-promoting, higher-priced foods, take advantage of sales on these products and stock up.

- *Just Pure Foods organic snack foods.* These vegetable-based, ready-to-eat snack foods are made from organic produce and whole foods that are low-temperature dried and sprouted to maximize enzyme and nutrient availability. Steer clear of the varieties with sweet ingredients, such as dates. My favorite is the organic Pesto Zucchini Chips.

- *Organic kale chips by different companies.* Kale is a nutrient-packed superfood, but conventional kale is sprayed with a pesticide toxic to the nervous system. Go organic and try eating organic kale chips as a healthy way to get more of this non-starchy, nutrient-packed vegetable in your diet. Many different companies make organic kale chips, but I suggest avoiding those that contain sweeteners as well as nutritional yeast, a potentially problematic ingredient to many. (A little background: Nutritional yeast is often grown on GM beet sugar or beet molasses. Even when it is organic or non-GMO, nutritional yeast is a highly processed product that contains free glutamic acid, which mimics the effects of monosodium glutamate or MSG, including causing headaches, facial pressure, and rapid heartbeat. It also can cause reactions in people with yeast overgrowth and some autoimmune conditions such as Crohn's disease.) A few examples to look for include Alive & Radiant Perfectly Plain and Hibiscus & Pink Peppercorn, Chocolatree Cheddar and Chipotle, and three varieties of Lydia's Organics Kale Krunchies.

- *Lydia's Organics crackers and chips.* Lydia's makes a line of raw dehydrated food products based on seeds, nuts, vegetables and fruits. Particularly helpful to many of my clients are its raw crackers—Italian Crackers, Green Crackers, Luna Nori Crackers, and Ginger Nori Crackers. These crackers are so densely packed with nutrients and fiber and relatively low in carbohydrates that just a few stave off hunger. They're especially valuable to take on trips. In some areas of the country, Lydia's also offers Rawkin' Pizza Chips, Rawkin' Carrot Chips, and Rawkin' Spicy Beet Chips, which aren't low carb but are very nutritious.

- *Go Raw Flax Snax and Raw Salad Snax.* Freeland Foods' makes Go Raw sprouted seed chips in flavors ranging from Simple Flax Snax to Pizza Flax Snax. Its latest creation is Go Raw Salad Snax, which is being test marketed right now. Salad Snax takes organic kale to a new level by mixing dried veggies in tasty combinations with a dressing made of organic apple cider vinegar, seasonings, and dried herbs.

- *Foods Alive Flax Crackers.* Foods Alive combines soaked and dehydrated organic golden flax seeds with seasonings and vegetables to make low-carb, flax-based crackers in flavors such as Mexican Harvest, Onion-Garlic, and Italian Zest.

- *Two Moms in the Raw Sea Crackers.* Two Moms in the Raw makes additional types of organic flaxseed crackers with herbs and kombu, a nutritious seaweed. Varieties that are available are Garden Herb, Pesto, and Tomato Basil.

There are plenty of organic and Non-GMO Project Verified varieties of corn chips, as well as substitutes for corn chips, such as bean and rice chips. You can buy these products and use them as occasional non-GMO "cheats" for parties. However, these products are heavily processed, contribute to carbohydrate cravings and weight gain, and are best avoided on a regular basis.

For those who can handle higher amounts of carbohydrates without adverse effects, the least processed snack foods are the organic crackers and Sticks and Twigs pretzels by Mary's Gone Crackers. They're made from organic, gluten-free whole grains and seeds.

Canned Foods, Condiments, and Soups

Canned and jarred foods, condiments, and soups are common items that contain hidden GMOs, food additives, and vegetable oils, so be choosy about the ones you buy. The following are what I consider to be the best choices in these areas of the store:

Tuna: When you need a little fast food, canned tuna can fit the bill. Many types of canned tuna packed in olive oil will do, but Wild Planet Foods is a standout in this category for several reasons. Its tuna is caught from pole and troll catch fisheries instead of the most common method of tuna fishing, longline, which results in large quantities of unwanted fish and animals, including threatened or endangered species, being accidentally caught. Pole-and-troll caught tuna is the most sustainable choice. Plus, Wild Planet has the highest amount of beneficial omega-3 fats and lowest amount of mercury and it doesn't taste fishy. Even many of my clients who don't like fish enjoy it. All of the varieties taste better than typical canned tuna, but for the best flavor, I recommend Wild Planet's albacore tuna packed in olive oil.

Olives, sun-dried tomatoes in olive oil, roasted red peppers, and artichoke hearts: These flavorful items make helpful additions to salads and other recipes. To avoid hidden GM ingredients or food additives, look for organic or Non-GMO Project Verified varieties, such as a wide variety of olives, sun-dried tomatoes in olive oil, and roasted red peppers by Mediterranean Organic, and canned Non-GMO Project Verified artichoke heart quarters by Native Forest.

Condiments: Avoid mayonnaise, which contains undesirable oils, and ketchup, which contains added sugar. Choose organic salsa instead, from companies such as Amy's Organic Kitchen.

In place of conventional soy source made from GM soy, look for San-J Organic Tamari Gluten Free Soy Sauce, which is Non-GMO Project Verified as well as organic. If you avoid soy, try Coconut Secret Coconut Aminos, a soy sauce substitute made out of organic raw coconut sap and sea salt.

Broth or soup: Search for organic varieties labeled gluten free by Pacific Natural Foods and Amy's Organic Kitchen. I also recommend steering clear of the varieties that contain corn and soy, even if they are organic.

Pasta sauce: Most of my clients avoid pasta sauces, which are too high in carbohydrates to control carbohydrate cravings or promote weight loss in many people. Some clients also develop aches and pains or digestive discomfort from eating tomato products.

If you and your family eat pasta sauce without any health troubles, be sure to go organic and select one with no added sugar. Eden Organic Pizza-Pasta Sauce is a good example of one with really clean ingredients. Another superb product is Mama Jess Garden Good 5-veggie pasta sauce. Made with organic tomato purée, carrots, sweet potato juice, onion, olive oil, red bell pepper, garlic, sea salt, and spices, this sauce is a fabulous way to sneak more vegetables into any kid's—or finicky adult's—diet. To eat even more vegetables, try it on spaghetti squash, a great pasta alternative.

Oils

The best types of oils to include on your shopping list are olive oil and coconut oil. Neither one is high in omega-6 fats, which contribute to immune system problems and inflammatory conditions in the body when eaten in excess. Olive oil is high in monounsaturated fats, and coconut oil contains easy-to-digest, medium-chain saturated fatty acids, making it a very stable fat to use in cooking. Both oils have a long history of safe use among humans. For the highest-quality coconut oil and olive oil, look for organic, unrefined, extra virgin varieties.

Tea and Coffee

If you drink tea, it's important to know that some varieties of tea actually have GM ingredients like soy lecithin and corn starch, and some tea bags are made from GMO corn. Tea also can be laden with pesticides. In a third-party analysis, more than 90 percent of the varieties of one popular brand of tea tested positive for pesticide residues exceeding the U.S. limits. To guard against this, look for organic, Non-GMO Project Verified tea from companies such as Choice Organic, Numi Tea, and Traditional Medicinals. These brands tend to be a bit more expensive than other brands, so watch for periodic sales and stock up. For the most current list of Non-GMO Project Verified teas, visit NonGMOProject. org.

The good news is coffee is GMO-free. The bad news is it, too, is often heavily sprayed with pesticides. No one wants to be sipping pesticides in their morning java, so seek out organic brands.

Though coffee and tea are not genetically modified, many ingredients that people add to their coffee and tea are. Wean yourself away from using sweetener in coffee and tea, and avoid milk products and highly processed milk substitutes such as soy milk. I recommend using canned lite or regular coconut milk instead. Organic varieties are available from Native Forest, Thai Kitchen, and Whole Foods' 365 brand.

Flours for Baking

Grain-based baking mixes often contain GMO ingredients such as sugar and cornstarch. Even if they don't, they turn very quickly to sugar in the body, so they are best avoided. For occasional baked goods, instead of grain flours, I recommend buying almond meal, blanched almond flour and/or coconut flour to bake with and using no to little sweetening, preferably just mashed up fruit such as banana or applesauce. Brands of almond flour on the market include Dowd & Rogers (blanched) California Almond Flour and Honeyville Blanched Almond Flour, and Trader Joe's unblanched almond meal. Organic coconut flour is available from companies such as Coconut Secret, Bob's Red Mill, Let's Do Organic, and Nutiva. You'll learn more about these flours in the next chapter and I'll provide some easy recipes.

As I mentioned in Chapter 8, it's best to avoid sweeteners in general. When you have a special occasion dessert such as a birthday cake, I recommend using coconut sugar (also known as coconut palm sugar), coconut nectar, grade B pure maple syrup, Non-GMO Project Verified honey, or unrefined cane sugar (Sucanat)—and preferably organic varieties of those sweeteners if possible. It's important to understand that fructose is the part of sweeteners that does the most damage in the body: It deranges liver function and promotes obesity and conditions such as type 2 diabetes and nonalcoholic liver disease. Coconut sugar and maple syrup have lower amounts of fructose, whereas agave nectar, which unfortunately is heavily used and promoted in the natural food industry, has a very high fructose content and is best avoided.

Refrigerated Foods

Salad dressing: Found in the refrigerated section in the produce department of some natural food stores, Tessemae's Salad Dressing is one of the few dressings that does not contain xanthan gum, a thickener that is derived from the common allergy-producing foods, wheat or GMO corn, soy, or milk, and can cause intestinal bloating in some people. Tessemae's Lemonette, Lemon Pepper, Cracker Pepper, Slow Roasted Garlic, and Zesty Chesapeake dressings are all Non-GMO Project Verified, and others are in the process of being verified. These dressings are made with olive oil, so they solidify when refrigerated. Be sure to bring a bottle out and let it sit on the counter for 30 minutes before you're going to use it. If you're pressed for time, try using the Lemonette dressing as a starter for a quick dip for steamed artichokes.

Hummus: Almost all pre-packed hummus on the market uses either soybean oil or canola oil. Both of these are the cheapest oils to use, are refined, and are almost always genetically modified. Even when non-GMO, they're often sprayed with lots of herbicide. Look in the refrigerated section for brands that use olive oil only. I found a local brand in my local health food store. If you can't find one in your area, invest in a food processor and quickly blend up your own with garbanzo beans, tahini, garlic clove, olive oil, salt, pepper, and lemon juice.

Guacamole: Guacamole made out of avocado, onion, garlic, jalapeno, cilantro, salt, and lime juice (and optional tomato), is even easier than hummus to make at home: You just mash it together with a fork. If you don't make it at home, you may be able to find Wholly Guacamole Classic and Wholly Avocado Chunky dip in the refrigerated section—or fresh-made versions by natural food stores with just real food ingredients. Skip any varieties that contain preservatives and additives.

TIPS FOR BUYING ORGANIC FOOD ON A BUDGET

It takes time, planning and effort, but anyone can move towards organic and keep his or her budget in line. Try these tips:

- **Pay attention to sales.** In large natural food supermarkets, there are more than 1,000 items on sale at any time, and many of them are organic.

- **Sign up for multiple store newsletters or circulars** or look for them in your local newspaper. Plan your shopping around organic items that are on sale that you most want and need, and then create meals from those items.

- **Capitalize on incredible one-day sales.** If you get email alerts about these super deals and make sure to go to the store on the day of the sale, you can save big.

- **Find coupons on the Internet.** Look on the websites of natural food supermarkets and click on the store nearest you to find weekly and/or monthly coupons. Also, study organic coupon sites, such as MamboSprouts.com, OrganicDeals.com, and SavingNaturally.com.

- **Check out the websites of your favorite food companies or join their social media pages** for coupons and special promotions.

- **Comparison shop to find the most economical organic items.** Within the same city, organic produce prices vary greatly. By shopping around, you'll get a general idea for which foods are cheaper at certain stores. Make sure to compare prices in stores' weekly ads.

- **Buy your most commonly consumed products by the case.** Some stores throw in a case discount and you can sometimes use coupons on top of that, even if the product is on sale.

- Stock up on organic non-perishable staples when there's a super deal.

- Be discerning. If you can't afford to buy entirely organic, choose wisely which items to pay more for. Know the "Dirty Dozen" deemed by the Environmental Working Group as the items that are best to buy organic. Or use this rule of thumb: buy organic fruits and vegetables that have thin skins, such as apples and berries. These foods tend to absorb the most pesticides and herbicides. Items with a thick skin or rind, such as avocados or citrus fruits, are less likely to be swimming in chemicals and can be bought conventional.

- Select produce that's in season as much as possible. When it's in season, it's much less expensive.

- Be the last to leave the farmers market. Many farmers will give special deals at the end of the day to sell their remaining produce rather than bring it back with them to the farm. For people on fixed incomes, it's also important to know that SNAP and WIC cards are accepted at many farmers' markets.

- Grow your own. Even if you only have a windowsill, growing potted organic herbs is a great strategy to keep down the cost of buying these overpriced items at stores.

Kelp Noodles: These low-carb, low-calorie noodles made by the Sea Tangle Noodle Company are made out of kelp, a sea vegetable that's rich in iodine and many other nutrients. Low-carb eaters can try the noodles in salads or add them to stir-fries or soups.

Raw Sauerkraut: Many practitioners recommend repopulating the gut with healthy bacteria. Eating small amounts of fermented vegetables such as raw sauerkraut, which contains probiotics, is one way to do that. Also, the tastes of various sauerkraut flavors give new, interesting ways to enjoy more vegetables in the diet.

Look for Farmhouse Culture Kraut, an organic and Non-GMO Project Verified product, in the refrigerated section. With flavors such as Classic Caraway Kraut, Garden Dill Pickle Kraut, and Horseradish Leek Kraut, you can enjoy these as side dishes, on top of burgers, or mix them with olive oil and shredded carrots to make a mellowed-out salad.

Salad Bar and Cold and Hot Prepared Foods

In natural food supermarkets that offer salad bars and cold and hot prepared foods, it's pretty easy to make a non-GMO salad at salad bars. It's harder—but not impossible—to find non-GMO options in the prepared foods sections.

Grabbing a salad from the salad bar may be more expensive than making a salad yourself, but the convenience is often worth the extra expense because it provides an easy way to have a non-GMO, and often organic, meal, especially for single people or those having a pressure-filled week. Steer clear of the usual GM produce impostors, zucchini, yellow squash, corn, and papaya. Then freely choose from a wide variety of fresh vegetables and fruits—everything from kale and walnuts, to spinach, cucumbers, radishes, carrots, and onions.

Beware that the prepared salads, dips, and salad dressings offered in salad bars are where GMOs and other unwanted ingredients are most likely to be. Read the ingredients, and look for dips such as hummus, prepared salads, and dressings made only with olive oil as well as dips, prepared salads, and dressings without GM produce items. To avoid salad dressings with GM ingredients such as canola oil and with sweeteners, you might need to dress your salad with olive oil and organic red wine or balsamic vinegar.

Among the prepared salads that are offered, you'll find that most contain soybean oil, canola oil, or a combination of olive oil and canola oil. If you're lucky, you can choose from a few made with olive oil only.

In the hot food bar, the very best deal by far is purchasing an organic rotisserie chicken. Avoid flavored varieties coated with ingredients like organic brown sugar, molasses, and cornstarch, and stick with "clean" varieties such as plain organic chicken with just salt and pepper, and occasionally organic rosemary and garlic, my favorite.

In the hot food line, look for steamed vegetables or vegetables sautéed in olive oil only. You can also usually find plain cooked brown rice.

As a general rule, steer clear of prepared soups. Virtually all that I have seen contain GM ingredients or additives I want to avoid.

When you strictly avoid GMOs, there aren't as many options in the prepared foods sections of natural food stores as it initially seems. It's my hope that if more people speak up and let natural food stores know they want more non-GMO and organic options in prepared foods, natural food stores will meet that demand, just as they listened to customers and now offer many non-GMO grocery products.

SHOPPING BY MAIL ORDER

If you have trouble finding certain organic or non-GMO products in your area or don't have a health food store near you, it's easier than ever to order products over the phone or Internet and have them shipped directly to your door. This strategy can work well for people who lack transportation, people who don't have easy venues for buying organic, grass-fed meats, and people from rural areas who want to stock up on organic non-perishable foods normally found in health food stores.

Many non-GMO and organic products can be ordered from websites such as ShopOrganic.com/ShopNonGMO.com and Amazon.com. Organic grass-fed meats and pasture-raised poultry also can be ordered online. Do an Internet search to find organic pasture-raised meat companies, or visit EatWild.com, click on the Shop for Local Grassfed Meat icon, then click on the Farms that Ship link.

One website some people like to order from is Vital Choice (Vitalchoice. com), a source for home delivery of fine wild sustainable seafood and organic fare. Vital Choice sells fish and shellfish that grow in the wild environment to which they are adapted and that are free of the antibiotics, pesticides, synthetic coloring agents, and genetically modified organisms used commonly in fish farms. Vital Choice seafood products are tested regularly by independent labs to make sure they are free of harmful levels of mercury and other industrial contaminants. They also have been tested for radiation.

Some of my clients order specialty products that are helpful for them on trips. One of these products is 100% grass-fed beef jerky chews by Sophia's Survival Food (Grassfedjerkychews.com). They are from cattle that are not fed GMOs and they don't contain sweet ingredients, soy sauce, or additives like most other beef jerky brands.

As when you shop in a grocery store, you need to be just as savvy a shopper over the phone or Internet. If you aren't sure about something about a product you're considering ordering, call the company or write an email and ask.

SHOPPING AT FARMERS' MARKETS AND DIRECTLY FROM FARMS

GMOs are hidden in so many foods in conventional and natural food stores that it pays to think outside the box of buying food only in stores. One of the best solutions for steering clear of genetically modified ingredients is to spend less time in grocery stores and more time at outdoor farmers' markets.

The Advantages of Buying Food at Farmers' Markets

There are countless benefits to buying food at farmers' markets. When you shop at farmers' markets:

1. **You get fresh, locally grown food.** At the farmers' market you purchase food that is fresh, ripe, in season, and recently picked, sometimes even that day. Most people realize how much better the produce tastes. By contrast, a lot of produce available in the supermarket is grown far from where you buy it. It is picked before it is ripe and sometimes artificially ripened later, then it is transported from different parts of the country or the world, and it can sit on the shelf longer than you might realize. The significantly greater length of time it takes from the farm until you buy produce in the supermarket affects its nutrient content, freshness, and taste.

2. **You help local farmers.** By eliminating the middleman of a store and purchasing food directly from farmers, you support farmers who grow food the right way by giving them most if not all of the profits from the sale of that food. In contrast, with produce sold in supermarkets, farmers get only a tiny percentage of the profits, and large corporations are the main ones that can stay in business in those circumstances. By purchasing locally, you do your part to help ensure that small local farmers can continue their operations to grow healthy food that's good for you

3. **You can obtain a greater variety of health-supporting foods.** By selling directly to consumers, farmers do not have to worry about their produce withstanding unnatural lighting, long trips, or temperature changes like supermarkets do. This means they can grow a wider variety of foods, including heirloom vegetables and other heirloom crops. Fresh produce is a key part of a healthy lifestyle, and exploring new varieties of produce makes for an exciting adventure. Heirloom foods hold historical interest, often have unique flavors, and sometimes have different colors than what we're accustomed to. Imagine purple carrots, yellow beets, and white eggplant that looks like a white egg, just like what it was named after! It's fun to explore these off-the-beaten-path foods.

4. **You may be able to buy organic food without organic prices**. Many times you can find food sold at farmers' markets that is grown organically—without synthetic pesticides and fertilizers—even when it isn't labeled as such. It costs a lot to receive organic certification, something most small farmers can't afford to do, yet some, perhaps many, don't use pesticides. The only way to know for certain is to ask the growers about methods used on their farm.

5. **You support your local economy.** Rather than benefitting major national corporations as is common when you shop in grocery stores, when you buy directly from farmers, you support small farms and help them stay in business. Those farms often create new jobs and hire more workers, further helping our local economies thrive.

6. **You are doing your part to protect the environment.** Instead of traveling 1,500 miles from farm to the supermarket as the average supermarket food does, food sold at farmers' markets only has to travel from the farms to the market to your table. Buying local, therefore, drastically reduces the amount of fossil fuels used in the production of those foods and the air pollution that goes hand in hand with more vehicle transportation; it's the eco-friendly choice.

7. **You experience more learning and sharing**. The more you make the farmers' market a regular part of your shopping routine, the more you can get to know farmers, see their passion, trust them and the food they're producing, and learn from them. When you know that they're supporting you, and they know you're supporting them, mutually beneficial relationships can develop. Farmers typically have a wealth of information about their product that they can share with you. They can explain the difference between various species of vegetables and often provide new ideas and recipes for the preparation of their produce or meats. When that happens, you feel even better knowing

you're using your money to support ethical small farmers and what they're doing.

What to Beware of When Shopping at Farmers' Markets

As beneficial as farmers' markets can be, it's important not to automatically assume everything sold there is safe and free of GMOs or pesticides. You still have to watch out for the usual GMO suspects and be an investigator, getting the straight scoop directly from farmers about what's in and on the food you're considering buying. For people who aren't accustomed to asking about what's in their food, this may take a bit of getting used to.

In most areas of the country, the main produce items to be leery of are zucchini, yellow crookneck squash, and fresh corn on the cob. If you see zucchini and yellow squash at a vendor's table, you won't be able to tell the difference between non-GMO and GMO zucchini or squash simply by looking at it, so you have to ask the grower. A typical question to ask might be: "Are this zucchini and yellow squash grown from non-GMO or organic seed?" If the farmer doesn't appear to know what a GMO is, you could try to educate him, or you could let it go and politely decide not to buy it. Farmers who are really against GMOs and are taking great steps to avoid them want customers to know that and will welcome giving you a detailed answer that assures you that the zucchini or yellow squash is non-GMO.

I never saw the big allure of sweet corn, but I have found that some clients, especially those who grew up in the southern United States, consider fresh sweet corn, also known as corn-on-the-cob, a special treat of summer. According to the Non-GMO Project, in 2011, Monsanto announced plans to grow genetically modified sweet corn on 250,000 acres, roughly accounting for 40 percent of the sweet corn market, and this GMO sweet corn started to appear on grocery store shelves, roadside produce stands, and in farmers' markets in the summer of 2012.[160]This type of corn is genetically engineered by Monsanto to contain the Bt insecticide and to resist weed-killing Roundup, so you don't just want to pick up any corn-on-the-cob without questions.

In an August 2013 blog post, certified holistic health coach Tracie Inman wrote that when she was at a farmers' market, she had already purchased half a dozen sweet corn, then she asked the vendor if it was GMO corn. The farmer's wife didn't know, but eventually found out from the farmer that it was GMO. Inman told the farmer she didn't want to eat that type of corn and politely asked for a refund, then she went on to a second vendor and found out that vendor, too, was selling GMO corn.[161] The fact is unless you ask before you buy, buying and eating sweet corn is a crapshoot, one that most non-GMO shoppers aren't willing to risk. The same goes for the corn used in corn products, such as corn tortillas and tamales. (Of course those who avoid corn or grains in general don't need to worry about this!)

Beyond avoiding GMOs at farmers' markets, you also likely want to know how the produce items are grown. Try asking, "Do you use pesticides on your farm?" or "What do you do to get rid of pests on your farm?" Pay attention to the answer you get and whether you trust what the farmer is saying.

In some cases, you might want to ask, "Can I come and visit your farm?" The farmer should be proud of what he is doing and happy to show it to you.

Sometimes small local farms will tell you they are Certified Naturally Grown (CNG) rather than organic. According to the Certified Naturally Grown website:

> To be granted the CNG certification, farmers don't use any synthetic herbicides, pesticides, fertilizers, antibiotics, hormones, or genetically modified organisms. CNG livestock are raised mostly on pasture and with space for freedom of movement. Feed must be grown without synthetic inputs or genetically modified seeds.

The description sounds like good, clean, non-GMO food production. However, when I asked one CNG rancher in my area some questions, I found that the produce he was growing was raised according to those standards and the cattle he was raising were grazing only on non-GMO native grasses, but the pigs he was raising were being fed genetically modified corn and soy supplemental feed! Beware that circumstances sometimes change on farms. Therefore, to avoid eating something you don't want, it always pays to ask farmers questions to learn what their current farming practices are.

In terms of vetting vendors for locally produced animal protein sources, know that ruminant animals such as cattle, bison, and lamb do best grazing on native grasslands alone, while chickens and pigs graze on grasslands but also require supplemental feed higher in protein that typically is from GM sources. Key questions to ask farmers and ranchers include:

- **"Are your cattle (or bison or lamb) all grass fed and grass finished?"**

  The answer to this question should be yes. Follow up by asking if the animals are fed alfalfa. If they are, ask if it is non-GMO or organic alfalfa, and if they say yes, ask how do they know it is.

- **"Do you ever give them supplemental feed?"**

  The answer should be no. If they say yes, ask what is in the feed. The answer will most likely be corn and soy, reason enough to avoid it.

- **"What do you feed your chickens or pigs?"**

  The answer is likely that the chickens and pigs graze on pasture and they're also given supplemental feed.

- **"What is in the supplemental feed you feed them?"**

  If the answer is corn and soy, ask if it's conventional corn and soy. Another way of asking this is, "Is the supplemental feed non-GMO or organic?" If they act like they don't know what you're asking, it's best to spend your money elsewhere.

Farmers' Markets vs. CSA Programs

It may not be convenient, or practical, to feed yourself and your family solely from the bounty of farmers' markets. But I recommend shopping there. When you are GMO savvy, farmers' markets are great places to not only help support local food production in your area, but also to make wise and healthy non-GMO choices for you and your family.

Before I leave this topic, it's important to mention another alternative that some people really like: Community Supported Agriculture (CSA); sometimes known as community-shared agriculture). If you have vetted a particular farm and like what it's doing, you may decide to join a CSA program with that food producer. CSA members or subscribers pay at the onset of the growing season for a share of the anticipated harvest. Once harvesting begins, they go once a week to pick up their weekly box of the most in-season offerings from that farm. To learn more about CSAs or find a CSA program near you, visit Localharvest.org/csa/.

Now that you've learned how to buy the most health-promoting non-GMO foods in traditional grocery stores, natural food supermarkets, farmers' markets and CSAs, it's time to start combining those ingredients, get cooking, and start eating! The next chapter will help you with basic food ideas and easy recipes.

Chapter 11:

Food Ideas and Recipes to Help You
Go Against GMOs

When you shop with non-GMO savvy and purchase clean non-GMO ingredients, it's easy to put together healthy non-GMO meals. You can use recipes you have and substitute non-GMO, preferably organic ingredients, or just get cooking creatively with the array of non-GMO real foods you buy.

I find that most of my clients don't use recipes on a day-to-day basis. They use them only for items they make infrequently, such as pancakes, a special occasion dinner, or a dessert. Therefore, although I include some basic recipes in this chapter, a lot of what I'll share here are assorted ideas for quick or easy non-GMO foods for both everyday and special occasions. Before each section of recipes is a section of background information and tips on how to use healthier ingredients you may not have tried before. This chapter is organized into the following sections:

- "Veg" Out
- Meaty Matters
- Fishy Matters
- Gluten-Free Grains and Beans
- Party Food
- Holiday Food
- Baked Goods
- Desserts

(I find that everyone needs to eat more vegetables, which is why I begin with the "Veg" Out section.) *All the recipes in this chapter are gluten free. Also, in the recipes, I list organic ingredients for the foods that are most important to choose organic, but I recommend using other organic ingredients as much as possible.*

Before you glance through the different sections, study the Non-GMO Substitutes list. To create non-GMO meals, use your regular recipes and make them non-GMO by substituting non-GMO, preferably organic ingredients in place of GM ingredients.

NON-GMO SUBSTITUTES

Substitutes for soybean oil, canola oil, corn oil, and cottonseed oil:
Unrefined extra virgin olive oil; coconut oil; avocado oil; organic butter; macadamia nut oil; sesame oil; or peanut oil (which isn't ideal but has a high smoke point and is better than a GMO oil)

Substitutes for "sugar" (almost certainly a combination of sugar from both sugar cane and GM sugar beets) and for corn syrup:
Coconut palm sugar; coconut nectar; 100% pure maple syrup; maple sugar; Non-GMO Project Verified honey; organic unrefined cane sugar; applesauce or mashed fruit; or mesquite meal

Substitutes for commercial chicken or beef broth:
Organic chicken or beef broth

Substitutes for soy sauce:
Non-GMO Project Verified San-J Organic Tamari Gluten Free Soy Sauce (Gold Label) or Organic Tamari Gluten Free Reduced Sodium Soy Sauce (Platinum Label); or Coconut Secret Coconut Aminos soy-free seasoning sauce

Substitutes for cornstarch:
Arrowroot or coconut flour (preferable because they're grain free); or Non-GMO Project Verified or organic cornstarch

Substitutes for corn tortillas and taco shells:
Organic blue or yellow corn tortillas and Non-GMO Project Verified 365 brand Organic Blue Corn Taco Shells

Substitutes for butter:
Organic, preferably organic pasture-raised butter; or organic coconut oil

Substitutes for milk:
Organic coconut milk; organic milk; or Non-GMO Project Verified organic unsweetened almond milk

Substitutes for cheese:
Organic and/or Non-GMO Project Verified cheese, preferably organic, pasture-raised cheese

Substitutes for conventional meats/poultry:
Non-GMO Project Verified and/or organic 100% grass-fed beef or lamb; grass-fed lamb from New Zealand; and chicken and turkey labeled Non-GMO Project Verified, organic, or organic, pasture-raised

Substitutes for farm-raised fish:
Wild-caught fish

Substitutes for zucchini and yellow squash:
Organic zucchini and yellow squash; locally grown zucchini and yellow squash grown from non-GMO seeds; or other varieties of summer squash, such as heirloom summer squash

FOOD IDEAS TO HELP YOU "VEG" OUT

Most people who come to see me for nutrition counseling are overweight or have cravings for carbohydrates or prediabetic or diabetic blood sugar levels, so the most common thing I do in my nutrition practice is teach people to reduce carbohydrates. On the most basic level, cutting the carbs involves avoiding starchy potato dishes and grain-based products such as noodles and rice, and substituting lower-carb, non-starchy, non-GMO vegetables, such as broccoli, asparagus, or spinach, in their place. Examples of simple vegetable-based side dishes that are easy to make include:

- **Roasted asparagus, roasted mushrooms, or roasted cauliflower coated in olive oil or coconut oil**

- **Steamed broccoli topped with organic butter or macadamia nut oil**

- **Stir-fried red or green peppers, onions, bok choy, and Napa cabbage in coconut or macadamia nut oil**

Another helpful strategy for eating more vegetables is to cut raw veggies (i.e., celery, carrot, and red pepper strips, cucumber slices, and radishes) ahead of time and have them in the refrigerator ready to eat at anytime. Use them with dips, on salads, or as sides with burgers.

You also can use non-starchy vegetables or vegetable-based products to make low-carb alternatives to normally carb-heavy side dishes, such as pasta, mashed potatoes, or rice. Try these low-carb, veggie-rich side dishes and see which you like best.

- **Spaghetti squash.** As the name suggests, this vegetable is a wonderful substitute for spaghetti, one that's considerably lower in carbohydrates and higher in nutrients. To prepare it, bake it whole or cut in half in the oven. Then remove the seeds from the center and use two forks to loosen the strands of squash, which look like spaghetti. Serve the "pasta" on plates and top with a homemade or organic gluten-free pasta sauce or pesto sauce, or organic butter or olive oil, garlic and herbs. An average spaghetti squash makes four to six servings and you can freeze leftovers. This alternative is best made in autumn and winter when spaghetti squash is in season.

- **Vegetable "spaghetti."** This is a low-carbohydrate, nutrient-rich pasta alternative that's perfect during spring and summer: Slice organic zucchini julienne style either alone or with other vegetables such as carrots, leeks and red peppers, sauté them in olive oil, and use the vegetables as a base for shrimp sautés or pasta sauce with meat.

- **Kelp noodles.** Made from water, the sea vegetable kelp, and sodium alginate (sodium salt extracted from a brown seaweed), kelp noodles have a non-fishy, completely neutral taste that picks up the flavors of whatever foods you use with them. They're available from the Sea Tangle Noodle Company. They're rich in iodine, which is essential for thyroid health, and they're almost calorie and carbohydrate free. This means they're a great addition to the diet of those who want to lose excess weight. They're also easy to use: Just open the bag, drain, use in salads, or add them at the last minute to soups or stir-fries. Try tossing them and sliced vegetables in sauces such as pesto or a non-GMO Asian sauce.

- **Shirataki noodles.** The key ingredient of this noodle replacement is glucomannan, a soluble fiber that keeps people feeling full for a long time. It's derived from the roots of the yam-like konjac plant. These uniquely textured noodles, available from Miracle Noodles, are thin, chewy, translucent, and gelatinous with almost no flavor by themselves, and they're carbohydrate and calorie free because they're made entirely of fiber. A drawback is they have an odd or unpleasant smell right out of the bag, which dissipates when they are rinsed well, simmered for a few minutes, and drained. Some people really like them, some people don't, but the angel hair variety generally is considered the best one to try. They can be added to broth, topped with sauce, or stir-fried in sesame oil with vegetables and a non-GMO, gluten-free soy sauce or soy sauce substitute such as Coconut Secret Coconut Aminos.

- **Mashed cauliflower.** With many different variations on this theme, mashed cauliflower makes a tasty low-carb alternative to mashed potatoes. The basic recipe starts with mashed steamed cauliflower, salt, and olive oil or organic butter. Variations include adding organic milk or unsweetened almond milk, cheese, different herbs, or roasted garlic.

- **Cauliflower "rice."** To make this quick dish, use a food processor with a shredding blade to shred chunks of a head of cauliflower until it starts to look like rice, then steam it for a few minutes in a bit of broth, or sauté it in organic coconut oil, butter, or olive oil about five minutes until done. Top it with an organic curry sauce, Asian vegetable and meat stir fry, or even grass-fed beef stew. One medium head of cauliflower will generally yield approximately six cups of cauliflower rice.

RECIPES TO HELP YOU "VEG" OUT

Here's a variation of mashed cauliflower with celery root and chives. Omit the chives if you're going to top it with gravy.

Mashed Cauliflower and Celery Root with Chives

1 medium head of cauliflower, cut into small florets
1 small celery root (also called celeriac), peeled and cut into ½-inch cubes
3 Tbsp. organic pasture-raised butter *or* 3 Tbsp. organic extra virgin olive oil *or* a combination of both
½ tsp. unrefined sea salt
1-2 Tbsp. chopped fresh chives

Set a steamer basket in a large pot and fill with water to just below the basket. Bring water to a full boil.

Add the cauliflower florets and celery root. Cover and steam until fork-tender, about 12-15 minutes.

Transfer cauliflower and celery root away from the pot, drain the water, and transfer vegetables back to the pot or into a serving bowl. Add the butter or oil and salt. Use an immersion blender to combine ingredients until smooth. Taste and add more salt if desired, then mix in chives. Serves 4.

Note: If you don't have an immersion blender, use a potato masher or transfer the ingredients to a food processor and process until smooth. You may need to add a Tbsp. of water, organic unsweetened almond milk, or organic chicken broth to get the right consistency.

_____

Here's a nutritious pasta substitute that makes an excellent accompaniment to baked fish or sautéed chicken.

Spaghetti Squash with Cilantro Pesto Sauce

1 medium spaghetti squash
2 cups loosely packed fresh organic cilantro, large stems removed
½ cup roasted macadamia nuts or pine nuts
2 garlic cloves, minced
2 Tbsp. lemon juice
1 Tbsp. lime juice
½ cup organic extra virgin olive oil
½ tsp. unrefined sea salt
2 Tbsp. chopped cilantro leaves for garnish

Preheat oven to 375° F. Pierce the spaghetti squash shell several times with a large fork and place in a baking dish. Bake for 25 minutes, turn the squash over, and bake until flesh is tender and yields gently to pressure, about 20 to 30 minutes more.

While the squash is cooking, strip the cilantro leaves from the large stems and set aside. Finely chop thin stems and place them in a blender or food processor. Add the nuts, garlic, lemon and lime juice, oil, and sea salt, and purée. Add the cilantro leaves and process until the leaves are coarsely chopped.

Once the squash is cooked, let it cool for 10 to 15 minutes, then cut it in half and remove the seeds and strings from the center with a spoon. Pull two forks lengthwise through the flesh to separate into long strands. Pile the "spaghetti" into a large bowl, add the pesto sauce, and mix well. Serve, and sprinkle with chopped cilantro leaves. Serves 4.

_____

Broccolette, also known as the trademarked Broccolini by Earthbound Farm Organic, is a green vegetable similar to broccoli but with smaller florets and longer, thin stalks. Stir-frying, then steaming/simmering with a flavorful broth is a quick way to cook broccolette.

Stir-Fried Broccolette with Garlic*

2 Tbsp. organic coconut oil, sesame oil, or macadamia oil
6 whole garlic cloves, peeled and cut in half
½ lb. organic broccolette (also called Broccolini)
¼ cup organic gluten-free chicken broth or vegetable broth
1 Tbsp. non-GMO Coconut Secret Liquid Aminos soy sauce
substitute or San-J Tamari Gluten Free soy sauce

Half or quarter the thicker stalks of broccolette lengthwise. Heat the oil on medium-low in your wok and add the oil. Add the garlic halves to the warm oil and stir-fry for a minute.

Add the broccolette, and stir-fry for 3 minutes, then add the chicken broth and non-GMO soy sauce or substitute, and cover the pan. Let the vegetable steam for 3 minutes. Remove the cover and continue stir-frying until the broccolette is crisp-tender and liquid has reduced down to your liking. Serves 2.

* Recipe adapted from a recipe for Garlicky Broccolette with Chile by Earthbound Farm Organic.

––––––––––

Research shows that artichokes are rich in antioxidants and minerals and are a wonderful source of silymarin, the active ingredient in milk thistle that helps protect and nourish the liver. They also help stimulate bile production, which helps digestion.

Steamed artichokes are served here with a simple creamy remoulade sauce. The hardest thing about this recipe is remembering to soak the walnuts in water overnight. To make the process easier, prepare the remoulade a day before, then simply steam the artichokes and serve with the sauce.

Steamed Artichokes with Walnut Dijon Remoulade*

1 cup walnuts
1 Tbsp. organic gluten-free Dijon mustard
¼ cup lemon juice
¼ cup organic cold-pressed extra virgin olive oil
1 large clove of garlic
Unrefined sea salt and pepper to taste
1-4 Globe artichokes

Soak walnuts in water and place in the refrigerator overnight. Drain and rinse. Place the soaked walnuts and the next five ingredients in a blender or food processor and blend until smooth and creamy. Store in an airtight container and use within 5-7 days. Make approximately 1½ cups.

To make the artichokes, use kitchen scissors to cut sharp tips off leaves if desired, cut off most of the stem, wash them in running water, and drain. Place them in a steamer basket inside a pot and make sure to add water to just below the steamer basket base.

Steam until a fork inserted into the artichoke bottom goes in easily— about 25 to 45 minutes, depending on the size of the artichokes.

To eat, pull off the petals and dip the white fleshy end in the remoulade sauce. Pull the soft, pulpy bottom portion of the petal through the teeth and discard the rest of the petal. Continue until all the petals are removed. Use a knife to scrape out and remove the fuzzy part, then cut the bottom (the artichoke "heart") into pieces, dip, and eat.

* Walnut Dijon Remoulade recipe courtesy of The Tasteful Kitchen restaurant in Tucson, AZ.

Variation #2: Steamed Artichokes with Lemon-Olive Oil Dipping Sauce: Steam artichokes as above. For a healthy dip made on the spot, combine Tessemae's Lemon Garlic Dressing and chopped fresh basil leaves—or olive oil, lemon juice, garlic powder or minced garlic, fresh basil, oregano, salt and pepper to taste.

Variation #3: Steamed Artichokes Dipped in Melted Coconut Oil:
Steam artichokes until done, then dip leaves in melted coconut oil. This is amazingly simple and so good!

Made with fresh in-season mangoes, this naturally non-GMO salad is a sweet summertime treat rich in vitamin E, vitamin C, and beta-carotene.

Mango Avocado Salad

> 2 mangoes, divided
> 1½ Tbsp. organic extra virgin olive oil
> ¼ cup fresh squeezed lemon juice
> 2 Tbsp. water
> ¼ tsp. dried basil (optional)
> Unrefined sea salt to taste
> 3 Tbsp. fresh organic cilantro leaves
> 4 cups organic romaine lettuce
> 1 medium avocado, chopped
> ½ cup organic red pepper, diced
> ¼ cup finely shredded carrot
> 2 Tbsp. diced red onion

To make the dressing, peel, slice and chop half of one mango. Place in a blender with the next five ingredients and half of the cilantro. Purée until smooth and pour into a serving container.

Combine the lettuce, avocado, red pepper, carrot, red onion and remaining cilantro in a large bowl. Peel, slice, and chop the remaining one and a half mangoes, add to the salad, and toss ingredients to combine.

Serve on individual plates and pour desired amount of dressing on each salad. (Cover and save unused dressing in the refrigerator to use on more salad the next day.) Makes 2 large salads or 4 side salads.

———

Here's a mostly raw dish that's quick to make on a hot summer day.

Avocado & Lime Cole Slaw*

3 cups shredded organic green cabbage + 1 cup shredded organic red cabbage
or 4 cups shredded Napa cabbage
1 Tbsp. minced red onion (*Optional*)
1 cup fresh organic cilantro
½ medium to large avocado
½ Tbsp. organic cold-pressed extra virgin olive oil
Juice of 1 lime
Celtic sea salt and pepper to taste
Pinch of ground coriander *(Optional)*
1-2 Tbsp. water if needed

In a large bowl combine the cabbage, red onion, and a tablespoon of cilantro leaves. Set aside.

Combine avocado, olive oil, lime juice, remaining cilantro, and seasonings, and blend until smooth. Add water if needed.

Pour into cole slaw and mix until dressing is well distributed. Refrigerate at least 20 minutes before serving. Serves 3.

* Recipe adapted from a recipe for Arizona Cole Slaw in my book *Going Against the Grain: How Reducing and Avoiding Grains Can Revitalize Your Health.*

———

This simple-to-prepare salad is bursting with the taste of summer from assorted seasonal vegetables and fresh basil.

Refreshing Summer Vegetable Salad

10 organic cherry tomatoes
10 organic pitted Kalamata olives
1 organic cucumber
¼ organic red pepper
1 cup organic spinach leaves
2 handfuls organic fresh basil
2 Tbsp. pine nuts
2-3 garlic cloves, crushed and minced
2 Tbsp. organic extra virgin olive oil
1 Tbsp. organic red wine vinegar
1 tsp. fresh lemon juice
Unrefined sea salt & pepper

Quarter the tomatoes; finely chop the olives, cucumber, and red pepper; and spoon the ingredients into a bowl. Slice the spinach and basil into strips, and mix them and the pine nuts into the other vegetables. Make the dressing by whisking together the garlic, oil, vinegar, lemon juice, salt and pepper in a cup. Taste, and add more lemon juice or salt and pepper to taste. Stir the dressing into the vegetable mixture, and serve or refrigerate for later use. Makes 4 side salads.

MEATY MATTERS

Clean animal protein is an essential part of most people's diets, and organic, 100% grass-fed meats are the types of meats our ancestors ate and the types we were meant to eat. As I explained in Chapter 10, compared to commercial meats from animals fed GM feed, grass-fed meats are far healthier and more nutritious. They have less total fat, saturated fat, cholesterol, and calories, and more vitamin E, beta-carotene, and vitamin C. With organic, grass-fed meats, there is less chance of getting something nasty like *E. coli*. Plus, grass-fed meats also have a much healthier fatty acid profile than grain-fed meats, and their taste is much lighter and "cleaner."

Differences in Cooking

When you switch to organic grass-fed meats instead of GM corn- and soy-fed commercial meats, it's important to know that because of their lower fat content grass-fed meats cook more quickly than commercial meats, so you have to be careful not to overcook them. In some cases, it makes little difference in how recipes come out. In others, it may take some minor adjusting in the beginning.

Generally speaking, for burgers, cook them less done than you normally would. For other cuts of meat, add moisture and prevent drying and sticking by cooking them at a low temperature in a sauce, using good-quality fat such as organic pastured butter or extra virgin olive oil when preparing them, or marinating them to tenderize them before cooking.

Organic chicken and turkey also are less fatty than their commercial counterparts. That means that they, too, come out best when you cook them in sauces, rub them or cook them in good-quality fat, or marinate them first so that they don't get dried out.

Different Ways to Prepare Good-Quality Protein

The key to having good-quality animal protein around is to cook your own meat or poultry for a meal and make extra for leftovers you can use to prepare fast-food meals a day or two later. This is a tried-and-true trick of the trade for all non-GMO eaters who eat meat.

On a cold autumn or winter day, there's nothing quite as comforting and mouth watering as *roasting an organic chicken or turkey breast or making homemade grass-fed pot roast*. The wonderful aromas permeating through your kitchen and surrounding rooms make the entire process comforting and gratifying. When you plan things right and take the time to cook this kind of homespun meal, you have delicious meat when it comes right out of the oven, and organic chicken, turkey or pot roast slices that make wonderful leftovers you can use in many ways.

Meatballs are another great item to bake for fast food a day or two later. You can make them with ground organic beef, lamb, buffalo, chicken or turkey and assorted finely minced vegetables and herbs, with or without almond meal as a filler. Serve them plain or topped with organic pasta sauce.

During hotter times of year or when you're too busy to take a few hours to cook, it's best to be your own short-order cook, something I do quite often. Make sautés or stir-fries with organic meat or poultry strips and vegetables—or try these other tips for preparing quick healthy protein:

- **Broil organic, grass-fed burgers.** These are ultra easy. Simply broil organic, grass-fed hamburgers, buffalo/bison burgers, or lamb burgers on both sides until done to your liking. Vary flavors by changing the types of meat and sprinkling different herbs or seasonings on them before broiling. Try Real Salt and pepper with: garlic powder or onion powder; herbes de Provence or Italian seasoning; or garlic powder and oregano, which are especially good on lamb burgers. Make beds of romaine or leaf lettuce and place the broiled burgers on top with sliced red onion and sliced tomatoes. To change the taste of hamburgers or buffalo burgers, top with a dollop of fresh guacamole or organic salsa or drizzle lightly with an herbed olive oil.

- **Broil steaks or chicken breasts or strips.** Try marinating organic, grass-fed steaks, organic chicken breasts, or steak or chicken pieces in olive oil, salt, pepper, garlic granules, and herbes de Provence or other herbs, then broil on both sides until done. This is a simple preparation technique anyone can do but it provides delicious, almost gourmet-tasting animal protein in less than 20 minutes.

- **Broil kabobs.** Broiling skewers of meat pieces or meat and vegetable pieces is similar but more versatile than the previous suggestion. You can make kabobs with pieces of organic chicken, grass-fed lamb, beef, or firm wild-caught fish alone, or alternate them with vegetable pieces—red onion, green, red or yellow pepper, cherry tomatoes, mushrooms, and organic/non-GMO zucchini or yellow squash. Cut the meat or have a butcher cut it into small pieces, which are the easiest and quickest to cook. Before cooking, marinate the pieces in an olive oil-based dressing so they stay moist when you cook them, then thread them on skewers.

A little trick when broiling: Remove the top broiler section of your broiling pan, cover the bottom with aluminum foil, then place the broiler section back on top of the bottom. This makes for easy cleanup when you're done broiling meats. All you have to do is clean the top broiler section of the pan. You simply wad up and throw away the aluminum foil that covered the bottom.

You can make variations of these broiled meat items by topping them with sautéed vegetables cooked in olive oil. Try:

- **Sautéed mushrooms**

- **Sautéed asparagus spears and minced garlic**

- **Sautéed onions**

I often sauté asparagus spears, mushrooms and garlic together and top an organic grass-fed burger with that combination, serve raw carrot sticks or cucumber slices on the side, and have fresh berries for dessert. It's a simple-to-make, nutritious meal. For the best health effects, always make sure to balance high-quality protein with vegetables.

MEAT & POULTRY RECIPES

A hearty, easy-to-make meal that's perfect for a cold winter day.

Savory Grass-Fed Pot Roast with Mushrooms

1 Tbsp. organic extra virgin coconut oil
1 small organic 100% grass-fed chuck roast (1½ - 2 lb.)
Unrefined sea salt and pepper to taste
1 medium yellow onion, minced
2 organic celery stalks, chopped
1 shallot, minced, and 4 garlic cloves, peeled and halved
2 tsp. dried French thyme leaves
2 tsp. dried rosemary leaves
1 cup organic gluten-free beef broth
8 oz. carton of button mushrooms, sliced

Salt and pepper the roast. Add oil to the bottom of a lidded, 10-inch, deep, heavy roasting pan and heat on medium-high heat. Brown all sides of the roast.

Place the onion, celery, shallot, and garlic on top of and to the side of the roast. Using your fingers, crush and sprinkle the thyme and rosemary throughout the dish. Pour the beef broth over the roast. When broth starts to bubble, cover the pan and reduce the heat to warm-low.

After an hour of simmering, remove lid, flip the roast over, and add the sliced mushrooms in the broth around the roast. Cover, simmer for 30 minutes, and cut into the roast to check for doneness, cooking for another 15 to 30 minutes if needed, depending on the thickness of the roast.

Turn heat off, sprinkle the meat with salt and pepper if needed, slice the pot roast, serve slices on plates, and ladle the broth and onion-mushroom-herb mixture on top of the meat. Serves 6.

———————

For a great brunch, try this easy-to-fix substantial meal.

Mexican Grass-Fed Beef Skillet*

1 lb. organic 100% grass-fed ground beef
1 tsp. + 2 Tbsp. organic extra virgin coconut oil
1-1/4 cups scrubbed and finely cubed organic Yukon Gold potatoes
1¼ cups chopped yellow onion
¾ cup chopped organic red peppers
4 garlic cloves, minced
1 small organic Serrano pepper, finely chopped
1 small organic Mexican grey squash or organic zucchini, finely cubed
1 tsp. dried oregano leaves
1 tsp. dried thyme
1 tsp. dried parsley flakes
½ tsp. ground cumin
1 small avocado, cut into slices
4 Tbsp. chopped fresh organic cilantro leaves
Unrefined sea salt and pepper to taste
½ cup organic salsa or more to taste
4 organic, pasture-raised large eggs *(Optional)*

Heat 1 tsp. coconut oil on medium in a large frying pan, and sauté ground beef about 3 minutes until slightly brown. Remove beef from pan and set aside. In a large skillet, heat 2 Tbsp. coconut oil, add the potatoes, and sauté until tender, about 4 minutes. Sauté in the onions and peppers for about 3 minutes, then add the garlic, Serrano pepper, herbs, and squash, and sauté for 2 more minutes. Mix in the ground beef and cook another minute or two until done. Turn heat to warm, and mix in salt and pepper to taste. Poach or fry eggs in another pan to desired doneness. Divide beef mixture onto four plates, and top each with chopped cilantro and a cooked egg. Arrange avocado slices on the side, and top with salsa or serve salsa on the side. Serves 4.

* Adapted from a family recipe for Mexican Beef Skillet by Mario Raso.

To offset the higher cost of grass-fed meats, buy less expensive cuts, such as lamb shanks, instead of leg of lamb. Try making grass-fed lamb shanks southern Greek-style—with lemon juice.

Greek-Style Grass-Fed Lamb Shanks*

4 grass-fed New Zealand lamb shanks
4 garlic cloves, peeled and sliced into slivers
4 Tbsp. organic extra virgin olive oil
Juice of 2 organic lemons
1 cup water
1 Tbsp. oregano
Unrefined sea salt and pepper to taste

Preheat oven to 350° F. Cut slits ½ inch wide and deep in several places on both sides of the shanks. Stuff garlic slivers into the slits, lengthening or deepening them as needed.

Add olive oil to the bottom of a lidded, 12-inch, deep, heavy roasting pan and heat on medium heat. Brown all sides of the shanks. Pour the lemon juice over the shanks. Sprinkle with oregano, salt, and pepper on both sides, then pour water in between the shanks. Cover the pan and place in the preheated oven. Bake for 30 minutes, then remove from oven, remove cover, and turn each shank to other side.

Cover the pan again and bake in the oven for another 2 hours, flipping the shanks to their opposite sides every 30 minutes. Check the meat for tenderness: meat should easily pull off the bone and have a wonderful aroma. If it doesn't, place back in the oven for another 15 to 30 minutes until done. Remove from oven, taste the jus, and season with salt and pepper to taste and additional lemon juice if desired. To serve, spoon the jus over both the shanks and side dishes. Serves 4.

* Recipe adapted from a recipe handed down from my Greek mother, Helen Smith.

Much quicker and easier than making lamb shanks is broiling lamb chops Greek style; it is by far the most flavorful way to cook lamb. This is a simple recipe that tastes gourmet. It works for both rib chops and shoulder chops. Rib chops are more elegant but much pricier. Shoulder chops require more cutting afterwards but are more affordable.

Simple Broiled Greek Lamb Chops

12 grass-fed lamb rib chops or 4 lamb shoulder chops
Unrefined sea salt and pepper to taste
Garlic powder
Dried oregano leaves
Lemon wedges to taste

Remove the rack of a broiling pan and line the bottom section of the pan with aluminum foil. Put the rack back on the pan and coat the top of the rack with olive oil. Arrange the rib chops or shoulder chops on the rack and sprinkle with salt and pepper and liberally with garlic powder and oregano on the top side.

Broil until the top side is browned, flip over, sprinkle the other side with salt, pepper, oregano, and garlic powder, and broil to desired doneness. Transfer chops onto four plates, pour natural au jus left in the foil-lined section of the pan onto the chops if desired, then squirt with fresh lemon juice and additional salt if needed before serving. Makes 4 servings.

Note: The time these take to cook sometimes varies depending on how thick the lamb chops are. When I broil at 450° F in my oven, it takes roughly 10 minutes to cook each side of average-sized lamb chops. Rib chops take a little less time.

Looking for foods that are easy to prepare and make great fast food a day or two later? Don't forget about meatballs. Here is an easy-to-prepare, veggie-enhanced meatball recipe made with grass-fed ground lamb.

Grass-Fed Lamb Meatballs Florentine*

1 lb. organic grass-fed ground lamb
3 garlic cloves, smashed and minced
¼ cup fresh organic baby spinach leaves, finely chopped
2 Tbsp. fresh organic parsley leaves, minced
¼ cup fresh organic basil leaves, minced
½ tsp. unrefined sea salt and more to taste if needed
¼ tsp. black pepper

Preheat oven to 350° F. In a bowl, knead together the lamb, garlic, spinach, parsley and basil until they are well mixed. Form into 1-inch meatballs, tucking in any herb or spinach pieces that are sticking out into the ground meat. Place in even rows in an 8 x 11½ x 2-inch baking dish. Bake on a medium rack for 20 to 25 minutes or until done to your liking. Sprinkle with additional salt to taste if needed. Makes 24 balls. Serves 4.

* Reprinted from my book *Gluten Free Throughout the Year*.

———————

Here's a simple, zesty flavored chicken that is easy to make.

Sautéed Organic Chicken Satay Strips

2 organic boneless, skinless chicken breasts, cut into stir-fry strips
¼ cup canned organic coconut milk
1-inch piece of fresh ginger root
1 tsp. garlic powder
½ tsp. unrefined sea salt
¼ tsp. pepper
1 Tbsp. organic unrefined coconut oil

Run the edge of a regular teaspoon down the skin of the ginger root to remove the skin, then finely mince it. Mix the ginger root, coconut milk, garlic powder, salt and pepper together in a deep-set bowl, add the chicken strips, stir well to distribute, let marinate for 10-15 minutes at room temperature, then stir again.

Heat the coconut oil on medium-low in a wok or deep-set frying pan. Add the chicken strips and ginger pieces from the marinade into the wok, and sauté 4 to 5 minutes on each side until done. Serves 2.

This is a favorite recipe of a close friend who feels as strongly about pure foods as I do. She eats an organic diet on a budget and combines this dish with organic vegetables that are on special.

Organic Chicken with Provencal Sauce*

4 (6 oz) organic skinless, boneless, chicken breast halves
¼ tsp. salt
¼ tsp. freshly ground pepper
2 tsp. dried herbes de Provence
1 Tbsp. organic extra virgin olive oil
2 Tbsp. organic butter, divided
2 cloves garlic, minced
1 cup organic gluten-free chicken broth
1 tsp. fresh lemon juice
Leaves from a few fresh organic thyme twigs (optional)

Place each chicken breast between two pieces of heavy-duty plastic wrap or parchment paper and pound as thin as possible, to less than ½-inch thickness, using a meat mallet, rolling pin, or small heavy skillet. Sprinkle chicken with salt, pepper, and herbes de Provence.

Heat 1 Tbsp. each of olive oil and butter on medium to medium-low in a large pan until butter melts. Add chicken, and cook 6 minutes on each side or until done. Remove chicken from pan and keep warm.

Add minced garlic to pan and cook 1 minute, stirring constantly. Add chicken broth and bring to a boil, scraping pan to loosen any browned bits. Cook about 4 minutes until chicken broth mixture is reduced down slightly. Remove from heat, add thyme, fresh lemon juice, and remaining butter, stirring until butter melts.

Serve the sauce over chicken and whatever vegetables you're having with the chicken. Season with additional salt and pepper if needed. Makes 4 servings.

* Recipe contributed by Susan Hughes.

———————

There are numerous at-risk GMO ingredients in typical Mexican cooking: corn, cheese, meat from animals fed GMO feed, and vegetable oils used in marinades, cooking, and salad dressings. By seeking out and buying organic or non-GMO ingredients—and using olive oil instead of canola, corn, cottonseed, or soybean oils—it's easy to make this versatile taco salad free of GMOs.

The chicken is very lightly spiced. If you like food spicy, add more cumin and some cayenne pepper and use a hot salsa.

Taco Salad with Broiled Chicken Strips

Chicken:
1-2 tsp. ground cumin
1-2 tsp. dried oregano leaves
½ tsp. garlic powder
½ tsp. onion powder
½ tsp. unrefined sea salt
Black pepper to taste
1 lb. Non-GMO Project Verified or organic boneless chicken breasts, pounded or cut thin
1 Tbsp. organic cold-pressed extra virgin olive oil

Dressing:
2 cups organic salsa
4 tsp. organic cold-pressed extra virgin olive oil
4 tsp. fresh lime juice

Salad:
4 handfuls organic, non-GMO corn chips, non-GMO bean and rice chips, or Mexican flaxseed crackers, divided
10 cups organic green or red leaf lettuce
5 green onions, chopped
1 pt. organic cherry tomatoes, halved or quarters (optional)
2 medium avocados, peeled, pitted, and chopped
2 oz. Non-GMO Project Verified or organic, preferably pasture-raised cheddar or Monterey Jack cheese, shredded *(Optional)*
4 Tbsp. chopped fresh organic cilantro

Preheat broiler. Mix the seasonings together well. Coat the chicken breasts in the olive oil, then in the seasoning mixture.

Cook on each side until no pink is showing and chicken is cooked through. Remove from broiler or grill and slice into ¼-inch wide strips.

In a large bowl, mix the salsa, olive oil, and lime juice together to make the dressing, and set aside.

Assemble the salads by putting several chips along the edge of 4 plates, then add the lettuce, green onions, and tomatoes in the center.

Top each salad with one-quarter of the chicken strips, pour ½ cup dressing evenly over each salad, sprinkle with avocado, cheese, and cilantro, crumble remaining chips on top, and serve. Makes 4 large salads.

Fishy Matters

Many types of fish are good sources of the beneficial omega-3 fats, EPA and DHA. Fish also is easy to digest and little fuss to make, meaning it should be a great answer to "What's for dinner?"

However, when considering sustainable food choices, none of us should ignore the fact that many types of fish have been hunted to near extinction and that some types of fishing accidentally catch unintended wildlife. When considering a safe food supply, it's imperative to know that most farmed fish are fed GM feed. We also can't ignore that the water in our rivers and oceans has become increasingly polluted. Plus, we still don't know how far reaching the radiation may be from Japan's Fukushima nuclear plant, which was damaged from a tsunami caused by a 9.0 earthquake that took place in March 2011. We all have to stay up to date on the latest information and make individual decisions about what is best for us and our families. So far, four rounds of tests on Pacific seafood products, including tests on salmon (pink, king, sockeye and silver), tuna, and Alaskan halibut, have found the fish to be safe.

For those reasons, I am providing a small number of foolproof fish recipes. They're good starter recipes because they are only for two people, don't taste fishy, and typically win over even people who say they don't like fish. They all are made with wild-caught fish that are not fed GMOs and that are listed as "Best Choices" or "Good Alternatives"—in other words, some of the most sustainable choices to select—by the Monterey Bay Aquarium Seafood Watch program.

Fish Recipes

Here is a light, easy-to-make entrée that is refreshing to eat on a hot summer day. A great thing about fruit salsa is it is a flexible recipe: You can make it according to your tastes and tolerances.

Baked Mahi-Mahi with Mango-Pineapple Salsa*

2 fresh wild-caught mahi-mahi filets
1 Tbsp. organic extra virgin olive oil or coconut oil
Ground coriander to taste
½ cup finely chopped fresh pineapple
½ cup finely chopped fresh mango or organic nectarines
1-2 Tbsp. minced green onions or shallots
3 Tbsp. minced organic cilantro or more to taste
1-2 Tbsp. diced organic red bell pepper
Ground coriander to taste
Cayenne pepper to taste (optional)
1 tsp. organic jalapeno, minced (optional)

Preheat oven to 400° F. Coat mahi-mahi filets and bottom of baking dish with the oil and sprinkle ground coriander over the fish. Cover the dish and bake until done, about 20 to 25 minutes. While the fish is cooking, mix together the salsa ingredients. When the fish is done, place it on a serving plate and top with salsa. Serves 2.

* Adapted from the Baked Mahi-Mahi with Fresh Pineapple Salsa recipe in my book *Going Against the Grain*.

―――――――――

This simple yet delicious recipe works with King Salmon (also called Chinook), coho (also called silver salmon), and sockeye salmon, which are in season at various times during the summer.

Roasted Wild Salmon with Dill

¾ lb. fresh wild salmon fillet
1 tsp. organic extra virgin olive oil or coconut oil
¼ - ½ tsp. unrefined sea salt
¼ tsp. black pepper
1 Tbsp. chopped fresh dill
1 tsp. grated lemon zest
4 (1/8-inch-thick) fresh lemon slices

Preheat oven to 450° F. Place fish, skin side down, on a foil-lined baking sheet coated with cooking spray. Brush fish with oil; sprinkle with salt and pepper. Sprinkle dill and lemon zest over fish; arrange lemon slices over fish. Bake for 10 minutes or until fish flakes easily when tested with a fork or until desired degree of doneness. Makes 2 servings.

When in doubt about what to make for dinner, go with the safest bet: meals based on naturally non-GMO foods. Try this simple, delicious recipe.

Broiled Lemon-Garlic Halibut

2 (6-ounce) Wild Alaskan halibut fillets
2 Tbsp. organic pasture-raised butter
2 garlic cloves, minced
¼ tsp. dried basil leaves
Unrefined sea salt and pepper to taste
1½ tsp. fresh minced parsley (optional)
2 tsp. lemon juice (optional)

Place halibut fillets skin side down on a greased rack of a broiler pan.

In a small saucepan, combine butter, garlic, and basil. Heat over low heat 1 to 2 minutes until butter is melted and garlic is softened and fragrant. Spoon melted butter mixture over each filet.

Broil halibut for about 10 minutes, or until it flakes easily when tested with a fork. Season with salt and pepper to taste, and sprinkle with parsley and lemon juice if desired. Serves 2.

Here's an ultra-quick recipe for one person, which is perfect for summertime because it involves no cooking.

Make sure to remove the olive-oil-packed tuna and sun-dried tomatoes from the refrigerator and allow them to sit on the counter for 15 minutes before you start making the salad. Doing this liquifies the olive oil and bring out its best flavor.

Mediterranean Tuna Salad

1 5-ounce can of pole-and-troll-caught, olive-oil-packed albacore tuna
2 organic sun-dried tomatoes in olive oil, chopped
1½ Tbsp. chopped fresh basil leaves
2 Tbsp. chopped Non-GMO Project Verified canned artichoke hearts
¼ tsp. garlic powder or garlic granules
Juice of ½ lemon
1 tsp. organic extra virgin olive oil
½ tsp. lemon zest
Unrefined salt and black pepper to taste

Place the tuna in a bowl and break it into chunks. Add the sun-dried tomatoes and artichoke hearts. Mix the lemon juice, olive oil, lemon zest, garlic powder, and basil together, pour into the tuna mixture, and mix. Season to taste with salt and pepper. Serve on a cup of salad greens. Serves 1. Double the recipe for 2 servings.

GLUTEN-FREE GRAINS AND BEANS

Quite a few of my clients experience their best health without grains or beans or they eat very few of them. Some, such as vegetarians, eat more of these foods to provide extra calories in place of meat.

For reasons I described in Chapter 8, all of my recipes and the food products I mentioned in Chapter 10 are gluten free. Try cooking Non-GMO Project Verified brown rice, organic, sustainably produced SRI rice from Lotus Foods, wild rice, and quinoa or beans, and creatively combine them with vegetables, herbs and seasonings, and good fats such as avocados, olives, nuts and seeds, or coconut oil. The following are a few basic recipes to give you ideas from which you can creatively adapt.

GLUTEN-FREE GRAIN AND BEAN RECIPES

Once the quinoa for this dish is made, this meal requires no more cooking and is easy to put together. If you remember to cook the quinoa the night before and refrigerate overnight, you can make a fast nutritious meal: Tossing the ingredients into the chilled cooked quinoa takes just a few minutes!

Organic Mexican Quinoa Bowl

1 cup organic red or white quinoa
½ tsp. unrefined sea salt
Juice of 2 limes
2 tsp. organic extra virgin olive oil (optional)
¼ tsp. ground coriander
¼ tsp. ground cumin
Ground black pepper to taste
2 medium green onions, white and light green parts only, thinly sliced
2 medium-large avocados, pitted, peeled and chopped
¼ organic red pepper, chopped
3 Tbsp. chopped fresh organic cilantro leaves
6 Tbsp. organic salsa

Bring the quinoa and water to a boil in a saucepan over high heat. Reduce heat to medium-low, cover, and simmer until the quinoa is tender, and the water has been absorbed, about 15 minutes. Scoop into a mixing bowl, and refrigerate until cold.

Gently stir in the green onion, avocado, red pepper, and cilantro. Mix together the lime juice, olive oil if desired, and seasonings, and stir the dressing into the quinoa mixture until well distributed. Mix 2 Tbsp. of the salsa into the quinoa mixture. Divide into four bowls and top each of the four salads with a tablespoon of salsa.

――――――――

Here's a quick, versatile breakfast recipe that's a convenient way to use up leftovers. Add organic, grass-fed meat or organic chicken pieces if desired.

Savory Quinoa Hash*

2 Tbsp. organic extra virgin olive oil or coconut oil
3 Tbsp. finely chopped yellow onion
1 cup cooked organic quinoa
3 Tbsp. finely chopped pecans
1/4 tsp. ground thyme
1/8 tsp. unrefined sea salt or more to taste
1-2 tsp. chopped organic parsley

Heat oil in a skillet on medium. Add the chopped onions and sauté for 30 seconds. Add the cooked quinoa, pecans and thyme, spread mixture across pan, and cook without stirring for 45 seconds. Then stir mixture and sauté about 2 to 3 minutes until golden brown. Take skillet off burner, mix salt into the mixture, serve, and sprinkle with parsley. Serves 2.

* Reprinted from my book *Gluten Free Throughout the Year*.

——————

This is an easy-to-fix dish for meat eaters who eat some higher-carb foods like quinoa and beans. To make the dish vegan, omit the chicken breast and cook the quinoa in organic gluten-free vegetable broth.

Mediterranean Chicken-Quinoa Salad

½ cup organic quinoa
1 cup organic gluten-free chicken broth
2 cups diced cooked Non-GMO Project Verified or organic chicken breast meat
½ cup organic garbanzo beans
3 Tbsp. chopped red onion
½ cup diced organic cucumber or organic English cucumber
10 organic cherry tomatoes, halved
¼ cup chopped Non-GMO Project Verified canned or marinated artichoke hearts
4 Tbsp. chopped fresh organic parsley
2 Tbsp. fresh lemon juice
2 tsp. organic red wine vinegar
2 Tbsp. organic extra virgin olive oil
2 garlic cloves, minced
Unrefined sea salt and black pepper to taste
¼ tsp. organic dried oregano leaves (optional)

Bring chicken broth and quinoa to a boil in a saucepan. Cover and reduce to a simmer. Cook for about 15 minutes or until all liquid is absorbed. Set aside to cool.

Combine chicken, garbanzo beans and vegetables in a large bowl, and stir in the cooked quinoa and parsley. Combine the lemon juice, vinegar, olive oil, garlic and seasonings in a small container to make the dressing. Pour dressing into the salad, and stir until well distributed. Serve at room temperature or chilled. Serves 2.

Below is a tried-but-true recipe that's been handed down in my family. It can be made with brown rice, but this one is adapted to use sustainably produced Madagascar Pink Rice. If you're just getting used to more vegetables in your diet, you can begin by using less spinach and gradually add more.

Greek Spinach and Rice

1 cup Lotus Foods Organic Madagascar Pink Rice
1¾ cups organic gluten-free chicken broth
2 Tbsp. organic extra virgin olive oil
1 small yellow onion, chopped
4 to 5 cups of organic baby spinach leaves (stems removed, if desired)
Juice of 1 small lemon
Unrefined sea salt and pepper to taste

Put the rice and chicken broth in a pan, turn heat to high until it starts to boil, then reduce heat to low, cover, and cook the rice until done, about 20 minutes.

Add olive oil to a deep-set frying pan, heat on medium-low, and sauté onions until soft, about 2 to 3 minutes. Add spinach leaves and quickly turn to lightly cook. (Spinach will cook down considerably from what it looks like when first added.)

Add onion and spinach mixture into cooked rice with lemon juice and mix well. Add salt and pepper to taste and squirt with extra lemon juice if desired. Makes eight ½-cup servings.

———

Simple to prepare, homemade hummus tastes much better than packaged hummus. Spread it on organic grain-free crackers or serve it with fresh veggie sticks, including jicama sticks.

Easy Homemade Hummus

    4 Tbsp. tahini
    4 Tbsp. fresh lemon juice
    2 cups cooked or canned salted organic chickpeas, drained
    2 garlic cloves, peeled
    1 Tbsp. organic extra virgin olive oil
    ½ tsp. unrefined sea salt or more to taste if needed
    1 Tbsp. water or more as needed

Process all the ingredients in a food processor or blender. Start with ½ tsp. additional salt and 1 Tbsp. water, and add more as needed to get desired consistency and saltiness. Makes 3 cups.

Note: If you use unsalted chickpeas, you will need additional salt, perhaps double the amount in this recipe.

Variations: For different flavors of hummus, add organic sun-dried tomatoes, roasted red peppers, or herbs.

———

To make super nutritious sandwich wraps, spread hummus on raw or lightly steamed collard leaves with chopped or shredded veggies and/or cooked chicken strips. You can make many variations. The recipe below uses steamed collard greens, which people tend to like more than raw greens, but you can easily substitute raw collard greens if you prefer.

Build-Your-Own Organic Collard Wraps
with Hummus and Vegetables

Organic collard greens, washed
Homemade or store-bought olive-oil-based hummus
Shredded carrots
Thinly sliced organic red pepper strips *(Optional)*
Sliced red onion pieces *(Optional)*
Chopped organic sun-dried tomatoes in olive oil *(Optional)*
Chopped avocado pieces *(Optional)*
Leftover broiled organic chicken strips *(Optional)*
Organic gluten-free Dijon mustard *(Optional)*
Organic goat cheese *(Optional)*

Flip each collard green leaf over so that the side with the prominent spine is facing up. Using a paring knife, carefully start to shave off the spine, starting near the bottom, where it begins to protrude most. Follow carefully along the spine, slicing away only the thick part of it, being careful not to cut through the leaves, which is what you wrap the sandwich in.

Steam the collard greens a few minutes until bright and tender, then arrange on a plate and use a paper towel to pat dry. Spread a few Tbsp. to ¼ cup of hummus on the inside of the leaf, then add veggies, chicken strips or other fillings to your liking.

Variation: Organic Collard Wraps with Chicken Strips and Veggies:
To make a bean-free wrap, omit the hummus and spread organic gluten-free mustard or an olive-oil-based, cheese-free pesto sauce, then fill with cooked chicken strips and shredded or sliced vegetables.

FOOD FOR PARTIES

Need to bring food to a party or make a spread of non-GMO food for a get-together of your own? You can do that non-GMO, and the party guests will never know the difference. Try these ideas for back-to-basics, naturally non-GMO, real-food light bites:

- **Assorted vegetable-based appetizers.** Think about vegetables to roast (such as garlic roasted asparagus spears or curry-scented roasted cauliflower), vegetables to stuff (such as organic celery sticks or Belgian endive spears), vegetables to top with toppings (such as cucumber rounds), vegetables to sauté (such as savory garlic sautéed mushrooms), and of course raw vegetable crudités with a dip. Or bring creative vegetable-based salads such as Avocado & Lime Cole Slaw or Mango Avocado Salad.

- **Protein-based appetizers.** What really transforms a spread of appetizers into a combination you can make a meal out of is including some hors d'oeuvres that contain slower-burning protein. For carnivores, meatballs made out of organic grass-fed ground beef or lamb often are perfect additions. Organic cheese or goat cheese fit the bill for some, and bean-based dips or nuts work well for vegans.

- **An all-in-one dish.** Especially if you're going to a potluck, make a dish that has protein and vegetables together. Then you're sure not to go hungry. One of my favorites to bring is colorful Shrimp (or Prawn)-Spinach-Artichoke Salad, the recipe of which I'll share later in this section.

- **Upgraded chips and dip.** Buy organic salsa, make your own guacamole with avocado, lime juice, garlic, onion, jalapeno, and fresh cilantro, or prepare hummus or homemade white bean dip. Serve with certified organic, Non-GMO Project Verified blue corn chips for higher-carb eaters, or better yet, serve with lower-glycemic non-GMO Beanitos Black Bean Chips, certified gluten-free Beanfields bean and rice chips, Foods Alive organic flax crackers, or thinly sliced jicama strips and assorted vegetable sticks.

- **Fresh fruit salad or fruit on a stick.** For a colorful, well-liked dessert, chop your favorite fruits and mix them together to make a fruit salad. Serve it in a clear glass bowl or a scooped-out watermelon or pineapple boat. Or thread equal-sized, ½-inch pieces of fruit onto skewers or party toothpicks. For a festive dessert, arrange equal-sized, ½-inch pieces of organic Granny Smith apple, peeled and sliced kiwi, pineapple cubes, and peeled and sliced banana on skewers and sprinkle with organic unsweetened shredded coconut.

PARTY FOOD RECIPES

Most dips for snacking or parties are made with milk-based sour cream, yogurt or cheese or soy- or canola-based mayonnaise, which likely contain GMOs. This delicious dip avoids GMO at-risk ingredients altogether. Serve it with Non-GMO Project Verified gluten-free chips, flax crackers, or fresh veggie sticks.

Creamy Macadamia Vegetable Dip

1 Tbsp. + ½ tsp. organic extra virgin olive oil, divided
2-4 Tbsp. water as needed
2 medium garlic cloves, minced
1 Tbsp. fresh squeezed lemon juice
1 cup macadamia nuts (raw or gluten-free, dry roasted)
¼ cup finely chopped fresh organic spinach leaves, stems removed
1½ tsp. minced red onion
1½ tsp. chopped fresh celery leaves
Unrefined sea salt to taste if needed *(Optional)*

Place 1 Tbsp. olive oil, 2 Tbsp. water, the garlic, lemon juice, and ¼ cup macadamia nuts in a blender or food processor. Grind, then purée until smooth. Add the rest of the macadamia nuts ¼ cup at a time, adding a Tbsp. more of water, grind then purée, and add a Tbsp. or two more water if needed to create a creamy texture. Pour purée into a bowl and mix in the spinach leaves, red onion, celery leaves, and ½ tsp. olive oil until well distributed. Makes 1 cup.

_____

Here's a fun, colorful item to bring to a party: a healthy change from mayo-filled deviled eggs!

Guacamole Deviled Eggs

12 hard-boiled large organic pastured eggs
1 medium avocado, peeled and pitted
1½ Tbsp. lime juice
3 Tbsp. finely chopped organic cilantro
1½ to 2 tsp. minced red onion
1 garlic clove, minced
1 Tbsp. minced jalapeno *(Optional)*
Unrefined sea salt and pepper to taste
Minced organic cherry tomato and red onion for garnish

Peel cooled hard-boiled eggs. Split the eggs lengthwise and scoop the yolks into a medium mixing bowl. Add avocado and lime juice to the egg yolks and mash, then add the rest of the ingredients and beat until well combined.

Use a small spoon to transfer filling mixture evenly between the egg whites. Garnish the top of each filled egg half with finely diced tomato and red onion. Makes 24 deviled eggs.

_____

This colorful dish is a real crowd pleaser at parties or potlucks. It's a ballpark recipe, meaning you can add a bit more of this or that, depending on your preferences and tolerances. It always comes out well.

The most sustainable choices when choosing shrimp, according to Seafood Watch, include Spot Prawns from British Columbia and the Pacific Northwest, Pink Shrimp from Oregon, and Sidestripe Shrimp from Alaska. If you prefer, make this dish with small pieces of organic chicken or with just vegetables. It's still tasty.

Shrimp-Spinach-Artichoke Salad

⅓ cup organic extra virgin olive oil
1-lb. bag of jumbo, peeled wild-caught shrimp or prawns with
tail-on, thawed
6 to 10 thin asparagus spears, chopped into 1-inch pieces
1-3 carrots, sliced
½ medium onion, chopped
¼ - ½ organic red pepper, chopped *(Optional)*
1 small shallot, chopped *(Optional)*
½ cup chopped Non-GMO Project Verified artichoke hearts
3 to 6 garlic cloves, crushed and finely minced
4 to 6 cups fresh organic spinach leaves (stems removed, if
desired)
2 to 3 Tbsp. chopped fresh organic parsley leaves *(Optional)*
Oregano to taste *(Optional)*
Ground coriander to taste *(Optional)*
Unrefined sea salt and pepper to taste
Juice of 2 limes and 1 to 2 lemons

In a wok, add extra virgin olive oil and heat on medium-low. Sauté hard vegetables—such as carrot slices, chopped fresh asparagus, and chopped onion—for 4 to 6 minutes until they're almost done. (You can add chopped red pepper about halfway through, if you're using it).

Add the shrimp and cook on one side until they turn pink, then turn each shrimp over and cook until pink on all sides. Then add the soft or quick-cooking vegetables: chopped shallot and garlic, artichoke hearts or sliced hearts of palm, and fresh spinach leaves. (The spinach shrinks when it cooks so add more than you think you need.) Add dried herbs and seasonings. Sauté until spinach is just barely cooked. Then take sautéed shrimp and veggies away from the burner and sprinkle with fresh parsley.

You can serve this hot, but to make as a cold salad to take to parties, transfer to a room-temperature Pyrex (glass) container. Add fresh lemon juice and lime juice. Allow to cool. (At this stage, you can take tails off shrimp and cut the shrimp into pieces—or you can leave them whole.

The shrimp with tails look elegant, but the shrimp pieces are easier to eat.) Once the mixture is room temperature, put lid on the glass container, and place in the refrigerator. The flavor is actually best half a day to a day-and-a-half later after marinating in the refrigerator. Taste before serving and add more lemon juice or herbs to taste if needed.

* Recipe reprinted from Shrimp-Spinach-Artichoke Salad recipe in my book Gluten Free Throughout the Year.

As an appetizer, low-calorie endive spears are typically filled excessive conventional cream cheese. When you get tired of weeks and weeks of heavy holiday food, try this light, endive-based hors d'oeuvre containing apple and fennel, two therapeutic foods for digestion, to get off to a healthy start in the new year.

Endive Stuffed with Fennel, Apple, & Walnut Salad

Zest of ½ lemon and ½ orange
1½ tsp. lemon juice
2 tsp. orange juice
½ tsp. organic gluten-free Dijon mustard
2 Tbsp. organic extra virgin olive oil
Unrefined sea salt and pepper to taste
½ large fennel bulb, sliced thin, and finely chopped
1 medium organic Gala apple, sliced thin, and finely chopped
½ cup toasted walnuts, finely chopped
2 Tbsp. organic dried cranberries
½ tsp. ground cinnamon
2 oz. organic goat cheese, crumbled (optional)
3 Belgian endive heads

Whisk the lemon and orange zest and juice, olive oil, and Dijon mustard in the bottom of a large bowl. Season with salt and pepper to taste.

Add the chopped fennel, apple, walnuts, and dried cranberries, and mix. Add cinnamon and additional salt if needed, and mix.

Slice 1" off the base of each endive. Arrange the spears on a serving plate. Lightly stir the salad and add the crumbled goat cheese if using, fill each leaf with the salad mixture until all leaves are filled, and serve. Makes about 2 dozen appetizers.

Pizza is a commonly eaten food laden with GMO cheese and toppings and a refined flour crust. If you occasionally eat organic cheese, try this homemade pizza. Eating this non-GMO pizza keeps blood sugar levels steadier than eating traditional pizza because the crust is made with low-glycemic almond flour.

Grain-Free Spinach-Mushroom Pizza

Crust:
2 large organic pastured eggs
2 tsp. organic coconut oil or extra virgin olive oil
2 cups blanched almond flour
¾ tsp. unrefined salt
1 tsp. dried basil leaves or Italian seasoning (optional)

Sauce:
6 Tbsp. to 2/3 cup homemade or jarred organic gluten-free pizza sauce, to your liking

Topping:
1 cup mushrooms, sliced
1 garlic clove, minced
1 Tbsp. organic pastured butter or organic olive oil
2/3 cup fresh organic spinach, chopped
¼ cup fresh organic basil, chopped
6 organic sundried tomatoes in olive oil, drained and patted dry (optional)
1 to 1½ cups shredded organic, preferably organic pas-ture-raised mozzarella cheese

Preheat oven to 350° F. Grease a pizza pan or cookie sheet to hold about a 9"pizza.

Beat the eggs in a medium mixing bowl. Add the other ingredients and stir. If mixture does not easily form a ball, add more flour by the tablespoon. Place the ball of dough in the middle of the pan and use your hands to press the dough into place until it's ¼ to ½-inch thick throughout the pizza and you form a crust along the edges.

Bake in the oven for about 15 minutes. While the crust is baking, sauté the mushrooms and garlic in the butter or oil just until soft, and salt if desired.

Spread pizza sauce evenly over the baked crust, and top with sautéed mushrooms, spinach and basil leaves, and shredded cheese. Return to oven, and baked for 12 to 15 minutes until cheese is melted. Using two spatulas, transfer pizza to a plate, slice into eighths, and serve. Serves 4.

HOLIDAY FOOD

GMOs lurk in most conventional holiday foods, but it's now possible to get non-GMO, organic versions of everything from eggnog to cranberry sauce to candy canes. However, based on my experience as a nutrition counselor, many people stray completely away from emphasizing blood-sugar-balancing real foods and end up experiencing cravings, weight gain, and deteriorated health during the holiday season.

To keep yourself strong and healthy so you can enjoy the holidays, I recommend that you limit sugar, be choosy about the foods you make, and go for quality more than quantity of food. Carb-laden side dishes, particularly sweets, baked goods, corn, mashed potatoes, and stuffing, make people feel bloated and uncomfortable and gain weight. Plus, preparing many different side dishes and coordinating them so they all come out when the main dish is done is difficult and stressful. To both make holiday meal preparation easier and feel better after eating holiday meals, select higher-quality organic ingredients whenever possible, prioritize the higher-carb, more labor-intensive sides that you and your guests most enjoy, and choose one or two to prepare.

If you are on a strict low-carb or Paleo diet, stick with the lower-carb substitutes such as Mashed Cauliflower and Celery Root that I covered earlier in this chapter. No matter what type of diet you follow, keep eating non-starchy vegetables as much as possible during the holidays.

The great news is the whole foods that most epitomize holiday meals are either naturally non-GMO or can easily be made non-GMO. That means you can enjoy seasonal pleasures without bitter health consequences. Here's a rundown of some common holiday foods and what to look for:

- **Roast Turkey and Gravy.** If you want turkey to serve as the centerpiece at Thanksgiving or Christmas dinner, be sure to special order an organic turkey several weeks before the holiday. If you're having a small group, order a much smaller and easier-to-cook organic turkey breast. You can make gluten-free, non-GMO gravy with organic cornstarch, but I prefer using grain-free arrowroot powder instead. Whisk 3 teaspoons arrowroot powder into ⅓ cup of water, and slowly whisk the mixture into boiling broth and drippings, stirring constantly while you add it.

- **Cranberries.** Festively ruby-red in color, rich in antioxidants, and tangy in taste, the cranberry is one of only three fruits native to North America that are commercially grown and an indispensable part of a traditional holiday dinner. To add holiday sparkle to everything from salads to wild rice dishes, seek out organic, Non-GMO Project Verified dried cranberries, such as those by Made in Nature. For cranberry sauce, buy an organic brand, or use organic ingredients to make a quick homemade version, which always tastes better than canned.

- **Mashed potatoes, yams, and other root vegetables.** Thanksgiving is a time to celebrate the autumn harvest, and the traditional vegetables of fall are root vegetables that grow in the ground, including potatoes, carrots, parsnips, turnips, rutabagas, sweet potatoes and yams. Baked sweet potatoes or yams are easy, popular, gluten-free Thanksgiving foods, and so are mashed potatoes. To prepare a more nutritious twist on mashed potatoes, try making mashed root vegetables with some orange and yellow root vegetables to give the mashed mixture a pale orange to yellow color.

- **Stuffing or dressing.** Stuffing or dressing can be made with herbs, celery, onions, and brown rice by itself or in combination with wild rice. It also can be made with no grain at all, such as with: chestnuts and vegetables; mushrooms, vegetables and nuts; or nuts, seeds, apples, and celery. Skipping the grain creates much lower-carb choices, which is better for controlling weight.

- **Wild Rice.** Naturally gluten-free, non-GMO wild rice is a true North American food, having been harvested, eaten, and prized by Native Americans for many centuries. It has a distinctive earthy flavor that's a natural for creating dishes, especially rice pilaf, that taste more gourmet than those made with brown rice.

- **Green Beans, Asparagus, Broccoli, or Brussels Sprouts.** At least one of these non-starchy vegetables is found on most holiday tables. For easy, yet special, non-GMO takes on these vegetables, try green beans almondine, roasted asparagus spears or roasted broccoli florets with garlic, and grilled Brussels sprouts that have been marinated in olive oil and herbs.

- **Simple desserts.** If you decide to have dessert (and some of my clients who are doing well on therapeutic diets decide not to), keep dessert easy to make and minimally sweetened. Try preparing crustless pumpkin pie with organic ingredients and pouring it into a well-greased pie plate. For a bit of texture in the pie filling, add chopped pecans to the batter before baking. One client who was caring for her ailing father didn't have the energy or time to bake a pie from scratch, so she set up an autumn sundae bar with organic coconut-milk-based vanilla ice cream substitute that guests could top with organic sliced pear, toasted pecans, cinnamon, and a drop or two of pure maple syrup. It was a hit with her dad and everyone else! The simplest foods are often the best.

HOLIDAY FOOD RECIPES

For smaller holiday get-togethers, roasting an organic turkey breast is easier and much more manageable than roasting an entire organic turkey. Here's one example of how to roast a turkey breast with flavorful fresh herbs.

Herb-Roasted Organic Turkey Breast

3 lb. fully thawed organic turkey breast
2 Tbsp. organic extra virgin olive oil
4 fresh sage leaves, chopped
Leaves from three fresh thyme sprigs, chopped
A few tsp. chopped organic parsley leaves (*Optional*)
Unrefined sea salt and pepper to taste

Gently lift the skin to expose the breast. Add the herbs, salt and pepper to the olive oil and rub between the breast and the skin. Place the skin back down and brush olive oil on the outside of the skin. Place the turkey in a roasting pan, roast in a preheated 400° F oven for 30 minutes, reduce the temperature to 325° F and roast until the middle of the turkey reaches 160 degrees, about 1 hour. Or cook according to package instructions. Place the turkey on a cutting board, cover loosely with foil and let it rest for 10-15 minutes before slicing.

———————

Roasting vegetables gives them a more gourmet taste. Roasting asparagus tones down the bitterness of asparagus and makes the flavor more mellow. It's common for people who don't like steamed asparagus to find that they like roasted asparagus.

Roasted Asparagus

1½ pounds asparagus
2 to 3 Tbsp. organic extra virgin olive oil or coconut oil
Unrefined salt and freshly ground black pepper to taste
Lemon wedges for accompaniment

Preheat oven to 375° F. Trim tough ends of stalks off the asparagus. Place asparagus in a shallow baking dish oiled with olive oil. Drizzle olive oil over the asparagus and turn asparagus spears around to distribute the oil. Bake asparagus until tender, about 10 to 25 minutes, depending on the size of the asparagus. Transfer to serving platter. Sprinkle with salt and pepper. Serve with a squeeze of lemon, if desired. Makes 6 servings.

For more convenience preparing your holiday meal, make this dish without the orange zest and parsley a day or two before the holiday, and refrigerate. On the holiday, reheat the dish and add the last two ingredients before serving.

Zesty Holiday Wild Rice

1½ Tbsp. organic extra virgin olive oil
½ cup chopped organic celery
½ cup chopped onion
2½ cups organic gluten-free chicken broth
1 cup Lundberg Farms Organic Wild Rice
½ cup chopped pecans
½ cup organic dried cranberries
1½ tsp. grated organic orange zest
3 Tbsp. chopped fresh organic parsley

In a medium saucepan, heat oil on medium-low. Sauté celery and onion about 5 minutes until soft. Add broth and rice. Bring to a boil, reduce heat to low, cover, and simmer for about 50-65 minutes or until rice is tender and the liquid is absorbed. Toast pecans in a 350° F oven for about 7-10 minutes until fragrant. Mix pecans and cranberries into wild rice, then fold in orange zest and sprinkle with parsley. Serve warm. Makes eight ½ cup servings.

I like pan-fried apples with cinnamon on winter holiday mornings with or without pancakes or homemade organic turkey sausage. This dish also can make a low-carb, Paleolithic substitute to sugar-sweetened cranberry sauce. However, the recipe is simple enough that you can make it anytime.

Pan-Fried Apples with Cinnamon

2 medium organic Granny Smith, Gala, Honeycrisp, or Pink Lady apples, chopped
2 Tbsp. organic pastured butter or organic extra virgin coconut oil
½ tsp. ground cinnamon
Unrefined sea salt to taste (*Optional*)

Melt butter or oil in a large skillet over medium heat. Add apples, stir, and cook for a few minutes. Add cinnamon and continue to stir about a minute more or until apples are tender. If you used coconut oil or unsalted butter, lightly salt to taste. Makes 2 servings.

In a rush during the holidays? Here's an easy-to-fix, refreshing, super-nutritious salad that's perfect to serve as a starter for a holiday meal or to bring to a holiday get-together.

Festive Kale Salad with Dried Cranberries and Toasted Walnuts

½ cup organic walnut halves or pieces
1 large bunch organic lacinato or dinosaur kale
1 organic orange
¼ cup organic extra virgin olive oil
2 Tbsp. orange juice (squeezed from ½ the orange)
1½ Tbsp. lemon juice
Unrefined sea salt and pepper to taste
½ cup organic dried cranberries

Begin preparing the salad two hours before you want to serve it. To toast walnuts, bake at 325° F about 10 minutes in the oven until they become fragrant and crisp. Wash and dry kale. Remove center ribs, slice the kale leaves into thin strips, and place in a large salad bowl.

Zest the orange. Place the orange zest, olive oil, orange juice, lemon juice, salt and pepper into a cup or small jar, and mix. Add the cranberries and toasted walnuts to the kale salad, pour the dressing throughout, and toss to coat thoroughly. Let sit on countertop for at least one hour before serving.

Slice remaining orange half lengthwise into thin slices, peel away rind, and chop orange slices into small pieces. Add orange pieces to salad before serving. Makes 4 salads.

For a break from tradition, try this colorful and nutritious twist on mashed potatoes.

Organic Mashed Root Vegetables

1½ lbs. organic rutabagas, peeled, cut into 1/2 -inch pieces
2 large organic carrots, peeled and thinly sliced
¼ small organic yellow onion, chopped
1 bay leaf *(Optional)*
1½ lbs. organic Russet potatoes, cut into 1-inch pieces
5 Tbsp. organic unsalted butter
4 Tbsp. organic gluten-free chicken broth
Unrefined sea salt and black pepper to taste

Cook the rutabagas, carrots, onion, and bay leaf in large pot of boiling salted water until almost tender, about 15 minutes. Add potatoes and continue cooking until all vegetables are very tender, about 15 minutes longer. Drain, and discard bay leaf.

Return vegetables to the same pot. Stir over medium heat to allow excess water to evaporate 1 or 2 minutes. Remove from heat. Add butter and chicken broth. Mash vegetables with a potato masher or immersion blender until the orange color from the carrots is well blended and the vegetables are almost smooth. Season with approximately ½ tsp. salt, taste the vegetables, then season with additional salt and pepper to taste if desired. Makes 6-8 servings.

With organic seasonal ingredients and no flour or cream, this decadent soup gets its creaminess from blended spring vegetables. It's a delightful starter for any holiday meal, but particularly for an Easter meal.

"Creamy" Asparagus Soup

1 lb. fresh organic asparagus
1½ tsp. organic extra virgin olive oil
¼ tsp. unrefined sea salt
¼ tsp. black pepper or lemon pepper
4 Tbsp. organic butter, divided
1 sweet onion, diced
5 organic baby red potatoes or 2 medium-sized red potatoes, peeled and diced
3½ cups organic gluten-free chicken broth
Salt and pepper to taste

Preheat oven to 375° F. Cut off and discard tough ends of asparagus. Place asparagus on a lightly greased baking sheet. Drizzle evenly with olive oil, sprinkle with salt and pepper, and roll to coat evenly.

Bake for about 5-6 minutes, turn the spears to the other side, and bake another 5 minutes or until tender. While the asparagus is cooking, melt 2 Tbsp. butter in a large pot or Dutch oven over medium heat, add onion, and cook, stirring frequently, about 3 minutes or until tender. Add remaining butter, stir until melted, add the potatoes, and cook, stirring occasionally for 3 minutes. Pour in chicken broth. Bring to a boil, cover, and simmer 5-7 minutes until potatoes are tender.

Chop asparagus into ¼-inch pieces. Add chopped asparagus to soup, and cook for 4 minutes, stirring occasionally.

Use an immersion blender to blend the soup until mostly smooth, but leave a few small vegetable pieces in the soup if desired. Season with salt and pepper to taste if needed. Serves 6.

Baked Goods

The secret to enjoying baked goods without the GMOs and without bitter blood sugar consequences is to use nut-based flours and coconut flour and other coconut-based products when baking. The following is a rundown of basic information about each of these ingredients. I'll cover more about sweeteners in the Desserts section to follow.

Almond Flour/Meal

The most commonly used nut-based flour is almond flour or meal. Almond meal and almond flour are both finely ground almonds and can be referred to as the same thing. In practice, however, almond flour is much more finely ground than almond meal, and most products labeled almond flour are made from blanched almonds (that have no skin).

For most recipes, you can use almond meal or almond flour, regardless of which is specifically called for in a recipe, and get good results. But the texture and taste will be different. Almond meal has a coarser consistency and tends to work better in breadings, cobbler toppings, and other types of recipes in which a coarser texture is desired. Blanched almond flour is a lighter, fluffier flour and is the preferred choice when a smooth looking, lighter-colored, and blander or milder baked good is wanted.

Almond flour is high in protein, high in heart-healthy monounsaturated fats, low in carbohydrates and sugars, and ranks low on the glycemic index, a rating system for how high different foods spike blood sugar levels. It's also highly nutritious, being a good source of vitamin E, manganese, magnesium, potassium, and fiber.

Research shows that eating nuts regularly confers many health benefits, including reducing the risk of type 2 diabetes, cardiovascular disease, sudden cardiac death, and macular degeneration. Researchers who studied data from the Nurses Health Study estimated that substituting nuts for an equivalent amount of carbohydrate in an average diet resulted in a 30 percent reduction in heart disease risk and an even more impressive 45 percent risk reduction when fat from nuts was substituted for saturated fats (which are found primarily in conventional meat and dairy products).[162]

Other big bonuses of almond flour are that it is moist, tastes rich and gourmet, and is easy to use. When eggs are used, baking with almond flour doesn't require adding thickeners or binders, such as GM corn-based xanthan gum, commonly used in many traditional gluten-free baked goods. When eggs cannot be used, you still can make pancakes and cookies by using egg substitutes and lightening the heaviness of almond flour with a lighter starch such as arrowroot powder. Almond flour's weight and fat content are so different from that of typical gluten-free flours that it's best to use recipes specifically developed for almond flour rather than trying to adapt recipes that use gluten-free flour.

Using different brands of almond flour/meal can make a difference in the way baked goods turn out, so experiment with different brands to determine which ones you like best. If you're gluten sensitive, look for Honeyville Blanched Almond Flour, a gluten-free certified brand, or Dowd & Rogers blanched California Almond Flour, which is gluten tested. I generally don't get good baking results when I use the more widely available Bob's Red Mill Almond Meal/Flour.

Trader Joe's makes an affordable (unblanched) almond meal that works well in some recipes. To save money, you can try making your own unblanched almond meal by whizzing small amounts of whole almonds in the food processor or a new coffee grinder until finely ground and then sifting for a finer consistency.

Coconut Flour and Other Coconut Products

Coconuts are the fruit of the coconut palm and have an amazing amount of food uses. Many coconut products can substitute nicely for common ingredients used in either traditional or gluten-free baking.

- **Coconut flour.** Coconut flour, which is fiber from the coconut meat after most of the oil has been extracted, can be a real boon for people who eat GMO free. Not only is coconut flour naturally non-GMO and gluten free, but it's also grain free and low carb, and it produces baked goods that are light, fluffy and moist. Baked goods made with coconut flour have a taste and texture similar to regular baked goods but don't prompt the blood sugar spike that regular baked goods do. To the contrary, coconut flour is so high in fiber (even higher than flaxseed!) that it holds down the blood sugar response.

  However, it has more fiber than any other flour, so it performs differently than other gluten-free flours.[163] That means that baking with it is a big departure from standard baking. A small amount of coconut flour is combined with several eggs to make baked goods such as cakes and muffins. If you haven't baked with this flour before, it's best to follow recipes specifically designed for coconut flour, such as the recipes in *Cooking with Coconut Flour* by Bruce Fife, N.D., until you become accustomed to it. For an egg-free dessert, mix coconut flour with chopped nuts, coconut oil, and coconut sugar to make a topping for fruit crisps or fruit crumbles. Organic coconut flour that either is gluten-free certified or has gluten contamination counter measures or testing procedures in place is available from Nutiva, Bob's Red Mill, Coconut Secret, and Let's Do Organic.

- **Coconut oil.** Coconut oil, an oil extracted from the flesh or meat of coconut, is a good dairy-free substitute for butter, lard, or margarine in baking. Coconut oil has a neutral flavor, is better than butter for "greasing" cake pans and cookie sheets, and is a very heat-stable fat. It's much healthier to cook with coconut butter than to heat omega-6 vegetable oils to high temperatures (and, in the process, create health-damaging free radicals and trans-fats).

  Coconut oil has numerous health benefits, including antiviral, antibacterial and antifungal properties.[164] It also is nature's richest source of medium-chain fatty acids (MCFAs)—also called medium-chain triglycerides or MCTs—types of fats that are easily digested and quickly burned by the liver for energy.[165] Look for organic, unrefined, extra virgin coconut oil, available from companies such as Nutiva.

- **Coconut milk.** Coconut milk is made by squeezing or extracting the oil-rich liquid from coconut meat.[166] The thick, creamy liquid makes a good non-dairy replacement for full-fat milk in recipes, or you can use lite coconut milk, or coconut milk that is thinned with water, in place of low-fat milk or non-dairy milk alternatives such as soy milk, almond milk, or rice milk. Look for organic unsweetened coconut milk from Native Forest or Thai Kitchen.

A very important tip to keep in mind: When using coconut oil, coconut milk, or coconut flour in a recipe, be sure to have all recipe ingredients that you're using, including eggs, at room temperature before preparing the batter. Using room-temperature ingredients will prevent coconut-based ingredients from chilling, hardening, causing lumps in the batter, and throwing off recipe results.

RECIPES FOR BAKED GOODS

On a cold weekend morning, warm up with these hearty grain-free, sugar-free pancakes. Serve plain, or with extra toasted walnuts, with walnuts and mashed banana, or with organic butter, a dab of pure maple syrup and cinnamon. Add non-GMO sausage to the meal to make a brunch.

Banana Walnut Pancakes

2 large organic, pastured eggs
½ banana
½ cup unsweetened organic almond milk or unsweetened coconut milk beverage
1½ tsp. organic gluten-free vanilla extract
1½ cups blanched almond flour
1½ tsp. arrowroot powder
½ tsp. unrefined sea salt
½ tsp. baking soda
½ tsp. ground cinnamon
½ cup chopped walnuts
Organic extra virgin coconut oil

Mix the first four ingredients together in a bowl. In a separate bowl, mix the almond flour, arrowroot, salt, baking soda and cinnamon together. Mix the dry and wet ingredients together. Finely mince the walnuts and mix them into the batter.

Heat coconut oil in a large skillet on medium-low heat. Drop a little less than ¼ cup batter into the pan and spread out batter slightly for each pancake. Flip pancakes when bottoms have browned, about 3-4 minutes, and cook for another minute or two. Add more oil to the pan and repeat with remaining batter. Makes 10 pancakes.

If you're allergic to eggs or looking for an alternative to help you avoid excessively eating eggs, try this tasty egg-free, grain-free pancake recipe in which chia gel (chia seeds soaked in water) is used as the egg substitute. You'll never know that the pancakes don't contain eggs.

Egg-free Almond Pancakes

2 Tbsp. organic chia seeds
6 Tbsp. water
¼ cup organic unsweetened applesauce
½ cup unsweetened organic gluten-free almond milk beverage
1½ tsp. organic gluten-free vanilla extract
1½ cups blanched almond flour
1½ tsp. arrowroot powder
½ tsp. unrefined sea salt
½ tsp. baking soda
½ tsp. ground cinnamon
3 Tbsp. chopped pecans
Organic extra virgin coconut oil

Place chia seeds in a small bowl, add water, and let sit 5-10 minutes until it's the consistency of a raw egg. Mix the chia-water combination, applesauce, almond milk, and vanilla together in a bowl. In a separate larger bowl, mix the almond flour, arrowroot, salt, baking soda, cinnamon and pecans together. Form a well in the center of the dry ingredients and pour in the wet. Mix together, but do not overmix.

Heat coconut oil in a large skillet on medium-low heat. Drop 1½ tablespoons batter into the pan and spread out batter slightly for each pancake. Flip pancakes when bottoms have browned, about 3-4 minutes, and cook for another minute or two. Add more oil to the pan and repeat with remaining batter. Makes approximately 16 pancakes.

A great combination of fruit, vegetable, nut, and coconut ingredients, this muffin is a healthy, fiber-rich addition to any breakfast or brunch.

Grain-Free Morning Glory Muffins

3 large pastured organic eggs *(at room temperature)*
3 Tbsp. organic unrefined extra virgin coconut oil, melted
¼ cup organic unsweetened applesauce *(at room temperature)*
2 tsp. organic gluten-free vanilla extract
¼ tsp. unrefined sea salt
¼ tsp. baking soda
1 tsp. cinnamon
1½ Tbsp. organic unrefined coconut sugar
¼ cup organic coconut flour *(at room temperature)*
½ cup shredded carrot *(at room temperature)*
¼ cup organic raisins *(at room temperature)*
¼ cup chopped pecans or chopped walnuts *(at room temperature)*
1 tsp. grated organic orange zest *(Optional)*
2 Tbsp. organic unsweetened shredded coconut *(Optional)*

Preheat oven to 350° F. Grease 6 muffin cups well with coconut oil. Mix together eggs, coconut oil, applesauce, and vanilla. Add in the salt, baking soda, cinnamon, and coconut sugar. Whisk the coconut flour into the batter until there are no lumps. Fold in the shredded carrot, raisins and nuts. Fill muffin cups with batter. Sprinkle with shredded coconut on top. Bake for 20 minutes or until a toothpick comes out clean. Cool on a wire rack, then refrigerate. Makes 6 muffins. Recipe may be doubled to make a dozen.

Here's a simple recipe for a grain-free, low-carb, low-glycemic biscuit that's a handy bread substitute. Try it with organic chicken and non-GMO, gluten-free gravy on top, or make a sandwich or open-faced sandwich with grass-fed pot roast slices, a poached or fried egg, or nut butter and apple slices. Make sure to have all ingredients at room temperature before you start mixing the batter.

Simple Grain-Free Biscuits

⅓ cup organic coconut flour *(at room temperature)*
5 Tbsp. organic coconut oil or organic butter, melted
4 large organic pastured eggs *(at room temperature)*
¼ tsp. unrefined sea salt
¼ tsp. baking soda
½ tsp. organic apple cider vinegar *(at room temperature)*

Preheat oven to 400°F. Line a large baking sheet with parchment paper. Mix the coconut flour, oil, eggs, and salt together. Add the baking soda, then the apple cider vinegar, and quickly mix to distribute throughout.

Drop rounded tablespoons of batter onto the baking sheet. Use the back of a spoon or your hands to spread the batter into rounded disc shapes 2½ inches wide and about ¼ inch thick. Bake for 11 to 13 minutes, until moist but cooked through. Cool about 10 minutes before serving. Makes 9 biscuits.

DESSERTS

As I explained in Chapter 8, there are countless reasons to wean yourself away from sugar and other sweeteners to promote optimal health. When you do, your blood sugar metabolism and overall health dramatically improve, your taste for sweetness lessens, and you appreciate the flavor of naturally sweet vegetables (such as carrots and sweet potatoes), fruit, and sweet spices (such as cinnamon).

Once you do this, you can much more thoroughly enjoy the best and easiest-to-make "dessert": fresh fruit at the peak of its freshness—or as a second choice, frozen thawed unsweetened fruit—by itself, sprinkled with cinnamon, or topped with unsweetened shredded coconut or coconut milk. Here are some examples of my favorite fresh fruit "desserts" generally organized from less sweet to sweetest:

- **Sliced organic strawberries or organic raspberries topped with shredded coconut** (a particularly good choice for sugar-sensitive individuals)

- **Slices of organic apple such as Gala, Honeycrisp, or Pink Lady**

- **Sliced organic white nectarines or peeled peaches sprinkled with cinnamon**

- **Organic Bing cherries or cubes of first-of-the-season organic watermelon**

- **Fresh pineapple cubes topped with organic unsweetened coconut milk**

We should be eating these types of desserts most of the time.

Of course in life, there are special occasions, such as graduations, holidays, and birthday parties, when special desserts are called for. Whenever possible, use mashed fruit such as organic applesauce or mashed banana to sweeten desserts.

When additional sweetening is needed, especially if you're making dessert for people who still have quite a sweet tooth, the best go-to sweetener in my opinion is coconut sugar or coconut nectar. Other non-GMO sweeteners that can be used on occasion are organic maple syrup, maple sugar, non-GMO honey, unrefined cane sugar, date sugar, or mesquite meal made from ripened, ground-up, naturally sweet yet low glycemic mesquite pods.

If you aren't familiar with coconut-based sweeteners, let me fill you in: Raw coconut nectar, a nutrient-rich sap from coconut blossoms, is a liquid sweetener that can replace honey or agave syrup in recipes. Unrefined coconut sugar, also known as coconut palm sugar, is made from evaporated coconut nectar, and can be used as a replacement for the same amount of sugar in recipes. TV show host Dr. Mehmet Oz lists it as a way to curb an addiction to regular sugar because coconut sugar doesn't cause the same blood sugar spikes as sugar.[167]

Both coconut nectar and coconut sugar do not taste like coconut but instead have a slight caramel-like taste. Either coconut sweetener is a good substitute for people who are avoiding fructose, honey, agave syrup, or all high-fructose sweeteners.

Fructose avoidance is a growing trend because some people have fructose malabsorption that causes digestive problems and many others avoid it because excessive fructose intake is implicated in the development of obesity, insulin resistance, metabolic syndrome, and diabetes.

Organic varieties of both raw coconut nectar and unrefined coconut sugar are available from Coconut Secret and SweetTree by Big Tree Farms. Organic, certified gluten-free coconut sugar is available from Nutiva and Shiloh Farms.

In the recipes that follow, you'll see that little sweetener is used. The only exceptions to that are the recipes for birthday cakes, which tend to be sweeter for the variety of people the cakes serve, and for chocolate, which is quite bitter on its own.

DESSERT RECIPES

The secret to this no-sugar recipe is using nectarines at the peak of their season when they're sweet, succulent, and juicy. I think the flavor gets even better when you make the crust and filling and refrigerate them overnight before topping with the sliced nectarines.

Grain-Free Fresh Nectarine Tart

Crust:
2 cups blanched almond flour
½ tsp. unrefined salt
2½ Tbsp. melted organic unrefined extra virgin coconut oil
1 large organic pastured egg

Filling:
1 cup organic coconut milk *(at room temperature)*
1½ small organic nectarines, peeled, halved, pitted and chopped
3 large organic pastured eggs *(at room temperature)*
1 tsp. organic gluten-free vanilla extract

Nectarine Topping:
2 organic nectarines (skin on), halved, pitted, and sliced
½ tsp. ground cinnamon *(Optional)*
2 Tbsp. fresh organic blueberries *(Optional)*

Preheat oven to 350 ° F. In a large bowl, combine the almond flour and salt. In a medium bowl, whisk together the coconut oil and egg. Stir the wet ingredients into the dry until thoroughly combined. Press the dough into a 9-inch tart pan or pie pan. Set aside.

Combine all the filling ingredients in a blender and mix well. Pour into the tart crust. Bake about 35 to 40 minutes until a knife inserted into the filling comes out clean. Allow to cool completely at room temperature. Then cover and chill in the refrigerator for a few hours or overnight.

Take the tart out of the refrigerator. Halve, pit, and slice the nectarines for the topping. If desired, sprinkle them lightly with cinnamon and mix. Line the nectarine slices around the outer edge of the tart, then work your way in to form an attractive, layered pattern on top of the tart. Sprinkle a small amount of fresh blueberries in the center for decoration. Makes 12 slices.

Slightly sweeter variation: Mix the nectarine slices lightly in prickly pear jam (from prickly pear concentrate) before placing them in the tart.

This is an easy-to-make, antioxidant-rich dessert made with low-glycemic coconut sugar. Serve it a la mode with a scoop of organic coconut-milk-based, vanilla frozen dessert and a few fresh blueberries for garnish.

Blueberry Cobbler

Filling:
2½ cups organic blueberries
2 Tbsp. organic unsweetened applesauce
2 tsp. organic gluten-free vanilla extract
3 Tbsp. unrefined organic coconut sugar
1 Tbsp. arrowroot powder

Cobbler Topping:
4 large organic pastured eggs
¼ cup organic coconut oil, melted
⅓ cup organic coconut flour
⅓ cup finely ground natural (unblanched) almond flour
¼ tsp. unrefined sea salt
½ tsp. Featherweight gluten-free baking powder
1 Tbsp. unrefined organic coconut sugar

Place blueberries in a 9-inch glass pie plate or baking dish. Add the applesauce, vanilla and coconut sugar, and mix carefully to coat the blueberries. Let it sit a few minutes before mixing in the arrowroot.

Preheat oven to 350° F. In a large bowl, whisk together the eggs and coconut oil. Combine the coconut and almond flours, salt, baking powder, and coconut sugar in a separate bowl, then stir it into the egg-oil mixture. Pour the batter over the blueberries, spreading it to the edges of the pan if necessary.

Bake 25-30 minutes until lightly browned on top and a toothpick inserted in the middle comes out clean. Cool for 10-20 minutes and eat hot, or for a sweeter cobbler, allow to cool, cover with plastic wrap, refrigerate, and serve cold. Serves 6.

––––––––––

With blanched almond flour, chopped walnuts, and organic coconut nectar, this naturally non-GMO, grain-free dessert is a low-glycemic alternative to apple crisp or apple pie made with refined white rice flour, starches, sugar or honey.

Grain-Free/Low-Glycemic Apple Crisp

Crisp Topping:
1¾ cups blanched almond flour
½ tsp. unrefined sea salt
1 tsp. ground cinnamon
½ tsp. nutmeg
⅓ cup coarsely chopped walnuts
2 Tbsp. unrefined organic extra virgin coconut oil (warmed so it is liquefied)
3 Tbsp. organic coconut nectar
1 Tbsp. organic gluten-free vanilla extract

Apple Bottom:
4 cups organic Gala apples, peeled, sliced thin, then chopped in half width-wise
1 Tbsp. organic coconut nectar
1 Tbsp. arrowroot powder
½ tsp. ground cinnamon

Preheat oven to 350° F. Mix the first five ingredients together. In a separate bowl, mix the coconut oil, coconut nectar, and vanilla. Stir wet ingredients into dry, then use your hands to combine the ingredients and create a crumbly mixture.

Grease an 8" by 11½", 2-quart Pyrex casserole dish. Mix the apples, coconut nectar, arrowroot, and cinnamon together and arrange in the baking dish. Crumble topping over the apples.

Place in oven and bake until dish is fragrant and top is brown but not burnt, about 18-20 minutes. Serves 12.

———————

Here's an easy way to make your own non-GMO dark chocolate.

Dark Chocolate Bark*

½ cup organic coconut oil
¾ - 1 cup cacao powder
½ cup unsweetened shredded coconut
1 tsp. organic gluten-free vanilla extract
¼ cup pure maple syrup (grade B recommended)
¼ cup chopped hazelnuts
1/8 tsp. sea salt

Melt the coconut oil on low heat and whisk in cocoa powder. Remove from heat and add remaining ingredients.

Pour into an 8½ x 6 ½-inch glass dish or pie plate and refrigerate until firm. Makes twenty 1½-inch square pieces.

* Recipe provided by non-GMO advocate Shea Richland from GMO Free Prescott.

This cake has a wonderful texture, is moist, and is versatile: You can top it with sliced strawberries or nectarines for strawberry or nectarine shortcake; frost it with a non-GMO frosting; reduce the vanilla and add ingredients such as cinnamon or orange zest; or enjoy it plain, as it is written below. My mother says all on its own, it's the best cake she has ever had.

Simple Delicious Cake

4 large organic pastured eggs
¾ cup unsweetened organic coconut milk
2 tsp. organic gluten-free vanilla extract
2/3 cup organic coconut sugar
½ cup organic coconut flour
½ cup blanched almond flour
¼ tsp. unrefined sea salt
½ tsp. baking soda

Preheat oven to 350° F. Grease an 8x8 inch cake pan.

In a large bowl, whisk together eggs, coconut milk, vanilla extract and coconut sugar. In a smaller bowl, combine coconut flour, almond flour, salt and baking soda. Mix dry ingredients into wet. Beat well until batter is smooth with no lumps.

Pour batter in cake pan. Bake for 22-28 minutes until a toothpick inserted in the center comes out clean.

Allow to cool for 10 minutes, then flip cake onto a plate, and flip it again so it is right side up. Allow to cool for 45 minutes or so. Serves 8.

A rich, decadent cake that tastes a lot like brownies when served plain or sprinkled with chopped nuts. For a more festive presentation, decorate the top with fresh organic raspberries and sliced organic strawberries.

Flourless Chocolate Walnut Cake*

2½ cups ground walnuts
½ cup unsweetened cocoa powder
5 large organic pastured eggs
1 cup maple sugar

Preheat the oven to 350° F. Oil an 8-inch nonstick cake pan and line bottom with parchment paper. Mix the ground nuts and cocoa powder with the eggs, one at a time, then slowly add the sugar, making sure everything is mixed well.

Spoon the mixture into the cake pan, place on the middle or upper oven rack and bake for 25-35 minutes, until a wooden pick inserted into the center comes out clean. Cool for 10 minutes or so, then turn out, remove lining paper, place right side up on a wire rack and serve. Serves 9.

* Recipe reprinted from my book *Going Against the Grain.*

Chapter 12:
Eating Out Non-GMO

Now that you've learned the GMO at-risk foods, how to select healthy non-GMO foods when shopping, and how to create non-GMO meals at home, it's time to apply your knowledge to eating out at restaurants and when traveling. This chapter covers the types of restaurants where you're most apt to be able to avoid GMOs, the main questions to ask restaurant owners, chefs, and managers so they can make non-GMO meals for you, and how to eat non-GMO during trips.

AVOIDING GMOS IN RESTAURANTS

At restaurants, you have much less control of which food options are, or can be made, non-GMO and organic than you do when you shop and cook for yourself. If you're like some non-GMO eaters who eat out infrequently, you may use eating out in restaurants as "mental health breaks" from the constant grind of strictly avoiding GMOs most of the time. If you do this, use the timeouts to focus on the atmosphere of the restaurant and the company you're with, and do the best you can at avoiding obvious GM foods, such as corn, soy, and sugar. Choose selections that emphasize non-GM fresh vegetables as much as possible.

However, if you're like other clients I have who are concerned about the health effects of GM foods or have allergies to GM foods, you want to strictly avoid all sources of GMOs when you eat out, just as you do at home. This chapter provides advice for steering clear of GM foods, but it's written knowing that you or some of your like-minded non-GMO friends may sometimes adopt lower standards when eating out, at least from time to time. If you are out with others who aren't as strict as you are, have a good attitude and be philosophical about it. Understand that we're all trying to maneuver through the challenges of avoiding GMOs in so many places, and we each have to make judgment calls and work with the information we're learning at our own pace.

Eating Out Non-GMO Basics

Because of what you learned in Chapters 6-11, you already have gained much of the knowledge you need to eat out against GMOs. Here are some key concepts for transferring the knowledge you learned in the shopping chapter to help you eat out non-GMO:

- *The foods that are GMO problem foods in grocery stores are the same foods that are likely GMO problem foods in restaurants.* For example, by knowing that close to 90 percent of the corn grown in the United States is genetically modified and that corn products in supermarkets are virtually all GMO (unless specifically labeled non-GMO or organic), you can assume all corn products in restaurants are GMO unless the menu specifically says they're organic and the owner confirms that with you.

- *Most processed foods contain GM ingredients, so just as it's important to avoid processed foods when shopping, it's important to avoid processed foods when eating out.* There are many different restaurants out there and some offer GMO foods galore and not much else. If you walk into restaurants that use mostly processed foods and try to get a 100 percent non-GMO meal, you might have to have a plain salad with no dressing and steamed non-GM vegetables—something many people don't want to do. To improve the chances of receiving a non-GMO meal that's worth going out for, look for restaurants that cook from scratch with fresh ingredients, not pre-packaged ingredients.

- *Cheap GM vegetable oils are used in virtually all restaurants.* This means canola oil or soybean oil especially, but sometimes corn oil. In many restaurants, olive oil is blended, thinned, or "cut" with GM vegetable oils such as canola oil. It's important to find restaurants that use 100% pure olive oil or other non-GMO oils such as coconut oil or sesame oil.

THE OIL ISSUE AT RESTAURANTS

Virtually all restaurants use GM vegetable oils in salad dressings and in cooking. Look for a restaurant that uses 100% pure olive oil. Your best bets are Italian, Greek, and Middle Eastern restaurants or high-end restaurants that have pure olive oil in their kitchens and can easily substitute it for the GM oils they typically use. Ask to be sure that the restaurant does not use an olive oil/vegetable oil blend.

General Guidelines about Different Types of Restaurants

Between 2012 and 2013, I ran a Pure Food Dinner program in the city in which I live, talked with many restaurant owners, and learned what is behind the curtain of numerous eating establishments. Though it makes sense given the ubiquity of GM foods in our food supply, this still came as a shock to me: *Almost all restaurants, even award-winning, high-end restaurants, use GM ingredients.* Just as many people use GM foods without realizing it, many dining establishments do as well.

Some restaurants, though, are more apt to have non-GMO options than others. To find eateries that give you more non-GMO options, it's important to first understand some general information about different cuisines.

Some cuisines are built around the very foods that are genetically engineered—i.e., Mexican is heavily based on corn and Asian is based on soy and small amounts of sugar. Also, both cuisines tend to use GM vegetable oils in recipes. Although you might be able to get a salad topped with fresh guacamole in a Mexican restaurant or vegetables stir-fried in sesame or peanut oil in an Asian restaurant, as a general rule, Mexican and Asian restaurants are best avoided because of the main food items that are emphasized.

GENERAL NON-GMO RESTAURANT SAVVY

The following are basic concepts to understand when eating out:

- **Mexican food is heavily based on corn,** a common GM food.

- **Asian food is heavily based on soy and some sugar,** which are common GM foods.

- **Italian, Greek, and Middle Eastern cuisines are based on olive oil,** which make them restaurants where it's easier to be able to order non-GMO meals.

- **A good first question to ask in any restaurant is**: *What kind of oil do you cook with and use in your salad dressings?*

On the other hand, Italian, Greek, and Middle Eastern cuisines are based on olive oil. Though you have to ask individual Italian, Greek, and Middle Eastern restaurants to be sure they use 100% pure olive oil, these restaurants, generally speaking, are much better bets to get non-GMO meals. Even if they usually use a vegetable oil/olive oil blend in cooking for the general public, they almost always have 100% pure olive oil on the premises and can sauté vegetables or wild-caught fish in it when requested.

When 100% pure olive oil is used in Italian restaurants, look for vegetable-based items, such as roasted asparagus, sautéed spinach, steamed artichoke, a medley of flavorful grilled or sautéed vegetables, or tasty salads.

In Greek and Middle Eastern restaurants, look for: hummus (a garlicky sesame-chick pea dip) and babbaghanoush (roasted eggplant dip with garlic and lemon) with sliced cucumbers; Greek salad or village salad (without feta cheese); sautéed spinach with garlic; roasted cauliflower; and green beans in tomato sauce (ask if the tomato sauce has added sugar). Higher-carbohydrate choices are Greek potato salad, roasted potatoes with olive oil and lemon, and skorthalia (whipped potatoes with olive oil and garlic): these side dishes are so dreamy, you can treat them like dessert! All three kinds of restaurants sometimes offer wild-caught fish and Greek restaurants may serve grass-fed lamb from New Zealand.

Beyond this general information about cuisines, know that cheap GM vegetable oils are almost universally used in salad dressings and cooking in the restaurant business, including in family-style restaurants, grills, restaurants in high-end hotels, and believe it or not, many farm-to-table restaurants, which emphasize fresh, local, and seasonal ingredients. That's why a good first question to ask when you're in any eating establishment is: "What kind of oil do you cook with?"

If the answer you receive is soybean, cottonseed, canola, or corn oil, or vegetable oil, margarine, or butter, all of those should be avoided. If the server or manager says they cook with olive oil, make sure it is not a blend of olive oil and some type of vegetable oil. Ask if they have anything that can be cooked without oil, or if olive oil or some other non-GMO oil such as sesame oil can be used. Even if you are not yet avoiding all GM-fed meat sources, which is a more advanced stage of going non-GMO, ordering, say, some commercial chicken cooked in 100% pure olive oil is a better choice than chicken cooked in GM vegetable oil.

Searching for the Most Promising Restaurants

Just as shopping at natural food supermarkets and farmers' markets improves your chances of getting non-GMO and organic food, searching for a promising restaurant is the best way to stack the deck in your favor to get a tasty non-GMO meal when eating out. Look for dining establishments that cook from scratch with real food ingredients, organic, grass-fed meats and wild-caught fish, and preferably organic and seasonal fresh ingredients.

Unfortunately, there isn't one website that lists all restaurants in the country with non-GMO menus. As of right now, finding the best restaurant for you depends on what type of non-GMO diet you follow.

Generally speaking, searching for organic restaurants on the Internet tends to reveal more vegan and vegetarian restaurant options while searching for grass-fed beef restaurants and farm-to-table restaurants tends to provide options with cleaner meat sources from animals not fed GM feed. (But you have to ask to be sure.)

**STEPS FOR FINDING RESTAURANTS
WITH NON-GMO OPTIONS**

To avoid hidden sources of GMOs, use the knowledge you learned about non-GMO shopping to ask questions in restaurants. The easiest way to get the information you need to order non-GMO choices—without appearing socially awkward in the restaurant with a group of friends or business associates—is to plan ahead. Follow these steps:

1. Get a copy of the restaurant's menu beforehand by picking up a copy at its location or visiting its website or Facebook page.

2. Study the menu, decide about which foods you need more information, and jot down questions to ask.

3. Call the restaurant during non-peak hours and ask to speak with the chef or manager about how certain foods are prepared, and if substitute ways of making foods, such as fixing a dish using pure olive oil, are possible.

I have used each of the following ways to search for the most promising restaurants to get non-GMO meals. Then I compare lists of the results I obtain from each of the searches. Try these different ways for finding your best bets for appropriate restaurants:

- **Search for non-GMO restaurants in your city.** If you're lucky, you might find that a non-GMO group in your area has done much of the searching for you and it may have a page that lists the best restaurant possibilities in your town to get non-GMO meals and how to order at each of those restaurants.

- **Search for organic restaurants in your city.** Searching for organic typically brings up names of restaurants that offer *some* organic foods. Even if "Organic" is in the name of a restaurant, understand that not everything on the restaurant's menu is organic and non-GMO. It's important to call or email the business—or ask questions in person—to find out what is organic and what isn't. For example, cheese typically isn't organic, but the salad greens and vegetables in the salad often are.

- **Search for farm-to-table restaurants in your city.** Farm-to-table restaurants usually mean the food used is fresh, local, and bought from farms. Searching for farm-to-table restaurants is a good way to find eateries that use more locally grown and seasonal produce items and sometimes locally raised grass-fed meats. But to avoid pesticides and GMOs, you still have to ask whether the produce is organic and whether the meats are organic and 100% grass fed and grass finished. In my experience, even many restaurants that use high-quality, local ingredients, organic produce items, grass-fed meats, and wild-caught fish tend to use GM vegetable oils in their cooking.

- **Search for grass-fed beef restaurants in your city.** Or look on Grassfedbeefrestaurants.com, a directory that lists establishments that serve grass-fed beef, bison and lamb, pastured pork and poultry, and other naturally raised meats. Though not every area is covered, many major cities are. Menus change frequently, so be sure to visit various restaurants' websites or call the eateries for their current menu selections to make sure the meat offered is 100% grass fed.

- **Search for gluten-free, food allergen-free restaurants in your city.** For many people who eat gluten free like me, searching under these terms is a mixed bag. Results often list restaurants that offer gluten-free baked goods, which virtually always contain GM or refined ingredients—exactly what you want to avoid.

  On the other hand, you can sometimes find a chat room or blog post about a particular restaurant that cooks from scratch and accommodates people with gluten intolerance and food allergies, including allergies to the main GM foods. To better ensure that you'll have menu options with fresher real food ingredients instead of processed gluten-free, GMO-laden ingredients, the best strategy is to find gluten-free restaurants that also appear on your non-GMO, organic, farm-to-table, and grass-fed beef restaurant searches.

What to Avoid and What to Look For on Menus

After you conduct searches and get a list of promising restaurants, the next step is to view their menus on their websites or Facebook pages. You can also stop by a restaurant and pick up a brochure-style sample menu to take with you to peruse.

As you're browsing the menu, look for obvious sources of GMOs that you want to avoid. Then look for entrées, such as a grass-fed burger, wild-caught halibut, or a quinoa-veggie bowl, that sound promising for being free of GMOs. If an entrée comes with a side dish that is made with GM ingredients (i.e., mashed potatoes made with commercial milk and butter), look at other side dishes that are offered on the menu (i.e. sautéed spinach or asparagus) that likely could be substituted.

Questions to Ask

Jot down questions that come to you. Here are some examples:

- Is your grass-fed burger organic and 100% grass feed (or grass fed and grass finished)? What ranch do you get it from?

- What kind of oil do you use in your salad dressing and in your quinoa-veggie bowl? Is there any soy sauce in it?

- Do you have 100% pure olive oil (not a blend) that I can use on my salad?

- Can I order the spinach or asparagus sautéed in pure olive oil in place of the mashed potatoes?

Then call the restaurant during off hours and talk to the chef, cook, or manager. This may seem like a hassle, but it's becoming easier because an increasing number of people in the restaurant business are aware that many people want to avoid GMOs or have allergies to GM foods.

The more you speak up and let restaurant personnel, especially chefs, managers, and owners, know about your strong desire to eat non-GMO food, the more they will not only make accommodations for you, but also begin offering more non-GMO choices on their menus. Depending on the answers and attitude you receive when you ask these questions, you can decide whether you feel comfortable and confident that the restaurant can safely meet your non-GMO needs.

Talking to the chef or manager beforehand is particularly important when you will be dining out for special occasions, such as birthdays and anniversaries. If you give chefs of good restaurants enough notice, you can often make arrangements for special non-GMO/organic (and gluten-free) entrees and even desserts, particularly if a large group of people will be coming for the gatherings.

AVOID THESE GM INGREDIENTS
USED IN MOST RESTAURANTS

Vegetable oil, canola oil, soybean oil, corn oil, cottonseed oil, cooking spray, and margarine (which are used but not typically listed on menus)

All **Corn** Products, including cornmeal, cornstarch, cut corn, corn tortillas, taco shells, and tamales

All **Soy** Products, including mayonnaise, soy sauce, tamari, tofu, miso, soy milk, soy cheese, and most veggie burgers and meat substitutes

Sugar and **Honey**

Papaya

Zucchini and **Yellow Crookneck Squash**

Butter, **Milk,** and **Cheese** (typically from cattle fed GM feed and that could be treated with rBGH)

Chicken, **Turkey**, **Pork**, and **Beef** (typically from animals fed GM feed)

Farm-Raised Fish (typically from fish fed GM feed)

OTHER FOODS THAT USUALLY CONTAIN
GM INGREDIENTS

Salad Dressing

Bread

Enriched Flour and Pasta

Fried Foods

Desserts, including Cake, Pie, Cookies, and Candy

Gluten-Free Baked Goods

Gluten-Free Desserts

Cereal

Ice Cream

Frozen Yogurt

Wine

Beer

Non-GMO Group Dinners

Speaking from firsthand experience, I can say that local non-GMO activist groups, particularly those with large groups of followers, have a unique ability to educate restaurants and influence them to offer more non-GMO meals. As the Pure Food Dinner Director of such a group for a year, I found that convincing restaurants that emphasized local and organic ingredients to agree to offer special non-GMO Pure Food Dinners on a particular night was easy because the restaurants saw the kind of following the non-GMO group had and wanted to work with it. When both the local non-GMO group in which I was involved and the restaurants that I worked with advertised the dinners, 25-45 people routinely attended these popular events.

The restaurant owners, managers and chefs were creative about the foods they offered and appreciated the extra business and good public relations the dinners brought them. We diners enjoyed non-GMO meals or several-course dinners with many organic ingredients. That made it a win-win situation for both the restaurants and the non-GMO group and its followers.

At each Pure Food Dinner I planned, I worked with the restaurant to offer two options: a vegan, gluten-free, non-GMO dinner, and a meat-containing, gluten-free, non-GMO dinner (if the restaurant served meat). Those two options accommodated most people who wanted to attend the dinners, including people who had the most common food allergies.

The following are sample menus from some of those dinners. Notice how vegetables are emphasized in all of the menus.

WHAT TO LOOK FOR ON RESTAURANT MENUS

For People on All Types of Diets:

All vegetables, except zucchini, yellow squash, and corn. Opt for organic varieties whenever they are available.

Unsweetened fresh fruits, except for papaya

For Meat Eaters:

Organic 100% grass-fed meats and wild-caught fish, either broiled with herbs or sautéed in olive oil

Organic, and preferably locally produced, pasture-raised eggs and chicken

For Vegans/Vegetarians and People Who Eat More Carbohydrates:

Quinoa, brown rice, and all types of beans except soybeans (but avoid these foods if they are cooked in commercial broth or prepared with vegetable oil, soy sauce, or milk products such as butter or cheese)

Examples for people who eat meat and vegetables:

Broiled Organic 100% Grass-Fed Burger with Homemade Guacamole and no bun, and an organic mixed green salad with red onion, cucumbers, & heirloom tomatoes, and olive oil and lemon juice

Seared Wild-Caught Alaskan Halibut Fillet with Sautéed Asparagus and Spinach in olive oil

Examples for vegans:

Grilled Portabello Mushroom or Eggplant with Homemade Tomato and Olive Sauce with Brown Rice

Veggie Spears with Red Pepper Hummus & Root Vegetable Salad

SAMPLE PURE FOOD DINNER MENUS
at a cook-from-scratch restaurant

Lamb Menu:

1st Course:
   Organic Greens with Organic Heirloom Tomatoes, Organic
   Cucumbers, & Organic Onions with Housemade Lemon
   Vinaigrette Dressing made with organic extra virgin olive oil

Main Entrée:
   Braised Grass-Fed New Zealand Lamb Shank with Lamb
   Rosemary Jus and Roasted Organic Root Vegetable Ragout

Dessert:
   Coconut Milk Brown Rice Pudding sprinkled with cinnamon

or

Vegan Option:

1st Course:
   Organic Greens with Organic Heirloom Tomatoes, Organic
   Cucumbers, & Organic Onions with Housemade Organic
   Raspberry Vinaigrette Dressing made with organic olive oil

Main Entrée:
   Seared Organic Eggplant with an Organic Tomato-Herb Sauce,
   Organic Red Pepper-Quinoa, and Roasted Organic Seasonal
   Vegetables

Dessert:
   Organic Cantaloupe Sorbet

ASIAN NON-GMO PURE FOOD DINNER BUFFET

Yin and Yang Salad: organic lettuce, kale, shredded cabbage, sugar snap peas, cilantro, other assorted vegetables and orange segments with Sesame-Ginger Dressing

Carrot Ginger Soup: made with organic carrot, celery, onion, garlic, and ginger

Asian Mixed Vegetable Stir Fry: Organic zucchini, carrots, mushrooms and other vegetables stir-fried in sesame oil and seasoned with Coconut Aminos, a soy sauce substitute

Rice Noodles with Spicy Almond Basil Sauce: made with Coconut Aminos, maple syrup, cilantro, chili flakes, and basil

Ginger-Infused Panna Cotta: made with organic coconut milk, ginger, maple syrup, and agar agar,
topped with Carmelized Orange Sauce: made with orange juice, maple syrup, and agar agar

HOLIDAY 4-COURSE DINNER MENU
AT A VEGETARIAN/VEGAN RESTAURANT

Starters:

Butternut and Red Lentil Soup &

Salad of locally grown organic mixed lettuce with roasted beets, oranges, walnuts, and organic apple cumin vinaigrette.

Choice of Main Courses:

Roasted Acorn Squash with Vegetable Risotto Stuffing and Organic Miso Mushroom Gravy

or

Casoulet Forestier – Mushrooms, white beans, carrots, onions and celery simmered in rich vegetable broth, placed into individual pots with locally grown organic mashed sweet potato topping

Served with sautéed pick-of-the-week local organic greens

Desserts:

All Organic Apple Crisp with Crème Anglaise made with locally raised non-GMO eggs, organic sugar, organic milk, and organic butter

or

Vegan Pumpkin Cheesecake with Coconut Cashew Cream

A LA CARTE NON-GMO MEALS
at a casual restaurant

Vegan Option:

Dinner Salad with mixed greens, cherry tomatoes, cucumber, and Olive Oil Citrus Dressing and

Grilled Vegetable Stack on Organic, Locally Grown Spaghetti Squash with roasted red pepper marinara

or

Wild-Caught Fish Option:

Grilled Wild-Caught Alaskan Salmon
on a bed of greens with cherry tomatoes, cucumber, with Olive Oil Citrus Dressing, and a medley of Grilled Vegetables

These menus show how innovative chefs can be when they are motivated to create non-GMO meals. Unfortunately, too few people let restaurant personnel know how much they want non-GMO food, so many chefs and owners don't understand the growing public demand for non-GMO choices.

To encourage more restaurants to offer non-GMO food options, it is up to us to let restaurant chefs and owners know of our strong desire for non-GMO and organic food. When enough of us speak up, restaurants will respond to what customers ask for, just as they did with gluten free.

A Note about Wine and Beer

Many people like to sip a glass of wine with a relaxing dinner in a restaurant from time to time, but few people realize that genetically modified yeast is used in the production of commercial wine and beer. To avoid the GMOs, seek out wine and beer labeled either "organic," "made with organic," or "Non-GMO Project Verified." To be labeled "organic" or "Non-GMO Project Verified," the wine or beer must be made with non-GMO yeast.

AVOIDING GMOs ON THE RUN

Completely the opposite of enjoying leisurely, relaxing meals is eating quick meals on the run. In the fast-paced world we live in, many of us have developed the habit of rushing through meals and plopping convenience foods in our mouths in a hurry. To eat against GMOs and take back our food and health, we have to break ourselves of this habit, find better alternatives on the run, and take more time to plan ahead.

The Hazards of Typical Fast Food

Fast-food restaurants offer foods that are sources of many GMOs as well as hidden sugar, salt, additives, and unhealthy fat. For all those reasons, we should avoid eating at these places.

When you find yourself in a situation where you have to eat fast food, know that the standards for what you eat there will inevitably be lower than what you can buy and make yourself. As of right now, there is not a viable supply of responsibly raised meats and dairy products from animals not raised on GMO feed, so there currently are no fast-food or large restaurant chains that offer meat from animals not fed GMOs. (As I mentioned earlier, getting GMOs out of animal feed is considered step 2 of kicking GMOs out of our food supply.) Also, just as the food products offered in grocery stores contain many sources of GM corn, canola, soy, and sugar ingredients, so too do virtually all the foods served in typical fast-food chains.

Chipotle Mexican Grill

To improve your chances of avoiding the major direct sources of GMOs when eating on the run, try eating at fast casual outlets that are making major steps to offer fresher, cleaner food. One national chain that is doing that is Chipotle Mexican Grill. As I explained in Chapter 1, in 2013, Chipotle became the first U.S. company to post labels on its website to let customers know which of its menu items contained GMO ingredients and it committed to phasing out the use of GM ingredients in its restaurants as quickly as possible. Chipotle previously used GM soybean oil in preparation of virtually all its foods, but during the last year, it switched to rice bran oil, a non-GM oil.

According to the ingredients page on Chipotle's website, which you can view online at Chipotle.com, the chain also uses: some organic ingredients, such as black beans, pinto beans, avocado, and cilantro; locally produced ingredients, including peppers, onions, jalapeno, and tomatoes; rBGH-free cheese and sour cream, with some of those dairy products from pastured dairy cows; and meat from animals not treated with sub-therapeutic antibiotics or added hormones. Those improved ingredients are all major steps toward a better quality of fast food. If you're a low-carb or grain-free diet eater, I recommend getting a salad with sautéed vegetables, meat, and guacamole. Other than the meat, you'll be avoiding all other GMOs—quite an accomplishment for busy eaters on the run. If you're a vegan, you can get a salad or brown rice bowl topped with beans, vegetables, guacamole, and salsa. Be sure to avoid the chips and the corn and flour tortillas, which all contain GMO corn and numerous additives. One other note: Chipotle's also is starting to offer an organic tofu-based entrée. You can learn more about it on its website.

Mediterranean Fast-Food Chains

Other good choices of fast-food restaurants are a few smaller fast casual restaurant chains, which offer Mediterranean food that specifically emphasizes the use of olive oil instead of GM vegetable oils. (Many Mediterranean fast-food restaurants don't.) One that does is Roti Mediterranean Grill, which offers build-your-own-meal entrées like Chipotle from a broad selection of vegetables, meat, and fish and better-for-you ingredients, including organic chickpeas, California Olive Ranch cold-pressed extra virgin olive oil, and Real Salt, an unrefined sea salt mined from Utah's ancient seabeds. When you order at the restaurant, steer clear of the breads; focus on the wide range of flavorful vegetables; and view its Allergen Chart to avoid sources of soy and gluten. The chain, which has restaurants in New York, Illinois, Washington D.C., Maryland, and Virginia, has significant plans for expansion in the next few years.

Another Mediterranean fast-food chain using olive oil and sesame oil is Zoës Kitchen, which has more than 110 locations in 15 states across the United States. Though it has more items made with soy and gluten ingredients than Roti, menu items such as its Mediterranean Tuna, Hummus, olive-oil-based Potato Salad, Roasted Vegetables, and Seasonal Fresh Fruit are all safe choices. You can learn more on its Nutrition & Allergen Information page at Zoeskitchen.com. (Just a note: Studying food allergen charts on a restaurant chain's website is a good way to identify hidden sources of soy, milk, gluten-containing products, and eggs, which are all common sources of GMOs. After you do that, the other two main sources of GM foods to ask about are canola oil and corn.)

Natural Food Supermarkets with Salad Bars

When you're short on time, you also can grab quick, healthy, GMO-free food at natural food supermarkets that have salad bars, such as at Whole Foods Market, Earth Fare, and some natural food co-ops. Avoid prepared salads made with vegetable oils and other GM ingredients. Instead, at the salad bar, select a wide variety of fresh, preferably organic vegetables, with additional ingredients such as nuts, quinoa, olive-oil-based hummus, or beans, and add animal protein sources, such as tuna, eggs, or chicken as needed. (Yes, the issue of protein sources from conventionally raised animals is a problem at these places, too. However, as I explained elsewhere in this book, many people need animal protein to keep their blood sugar levels stable to prevent sugar cravings and avoid eating blood-sugar- and insulin-spiking sugar and grain products that lead to countless health problems. In some natural food stores, you can buy an Epic organic, grass-fed lamb bar—or carry a bar with you and use that as a clean animal protein source with which to supplement the salad.)

Homemade Fast Food

To avoid being forced to visit fast-food restaurants without thought, the best solution is to plan ahead and make your own fast food by preparing larger-than-you-need amounts of foods for dinners. Here are some examples:

- Roast an organic, pasture-raised pot roast on a Sunday, eat it and save leftover pot roast and vegetables to reheat for future meals, or use the meat to top salads.

- Make a big pot of non-GMO, organic soup or a large stir-fry and have leftovers to heat up later in the week. To take hot foods with you to work, invest in a Thermos.

- Broil organic chicken or grass-fed lamb or beef kabobs, have some for dinner, then cut up the leftover meat and kabob vegetables (usually red onion, peppers and mushrooms), and reheat a day later, or add them cold to salads.

Also, don't forget to routinely get in the habit of carrying snacks. Nuts work especially well for short trips away from home.

Avoiding GMOs At Parties

If you are invited to a party, you may want to attend but feel certain that GM ingredients will be in most of the foods offered. You need to weigh how much you want to relax your standards during certain social situations versus how much you want to continue to eat strictly non-GMO. For staying strictly non-GMO at parties, try these tips:

- **Think before going to a party.** Talk to the host several days before the party, tell him or her that you are on a special diet, and politely ask what types of foods will be served. If the host isn't knowledgeable or accommodating, offer to bring a dish of your own—the main way to be sure you'll have non-GMO food to eat.

- **Bring an all-in-one dish.** When preparing an item for potlucks or parties, make one that has protein and vegetables together. Even if other foods aren't safe to eat, you can sustain yourself with the complete meal that you brought. Examples include: a large salad with broiled organic chicken strips, toasted almonds and pieces of organic nectarine; the Shrimp-Spinach-Artichoke Salad whose recipe was included in Chapter 11; or for vegetarians, a large salad with beans, onions, peppers, salsa, avocado, optional organic cheese, and a homemade lime vinaigrette dressing.

- **Eat before the party.** If you didn't talk with the host ahead of time or bring your own dish, make sure to eat some protein, such as leftover organic chicken or grass-fed pot roast slices, before you go to the party. The protein will keep you strong and satiated. Then look for veggie sticks or fruit pieces to nibble on at the party.

- **If not an all-in-one dish, bring an appetizer.** Make your own non-GMO dip and serve it with fresh vegetable crudités and non-GMO, organic chips. Or bring organic cheese and fresh fruit, or a large bowl of dry-roasted nuts. Though you may be paying more to buy these foods, you can feel good about providing the crowd and yourself something other than the usual GMO-laden, pesticide-laden party fare.

AVOIDING GMOS WHEN TRAVELING

When you travel, you experience a break from your regular routine and explore new, exciting environments. The unfortunate parts of traveling are you don't have the creature comforts of home and traveling is more hectic than it used to be.

General Tips for Non-GMO Traveling

Whether you're taking a road trip or flying to your destination, unexpected curves can happen, even on short trips. That means it's more important than ever to be prepared and plan ahead. Try these bottom-line tips to enjoy safe, pleasurable, non-GMO trips:

- **Always carry your own snacks.** Meal and snack service has been cut on most airplane flights, and virtually all of the food sold in airports and fast-food outlets, or on trains, contains GMOs or other unhealthy ingredients. That means it's essential to take your own non-GMO/ organic food. Virtually any non-GMO food will work in a pinch to give you temporary energy. But to keep yourself well nourished and strong for the extra time and effort involved in traveling, concentrate on giving yourself mini-meals that provide protein, healthful fat, and unrefined carbohydrates—i.e, nuts and an apple, organic grass-fed beef jerky pieces and carrot sticks, or a non-GMO food bar that contains protein.

- **Use a cooler when possible.** For road trips, pack a small cooler and some cold packs and take perishable foods on the road with you—i.e., hard-boiled organic eggs, chilled watermelon pieces, and homemade guacamole or olive-oil-based hummus with veggie sticks. Carrying perishable foods with you is a great way to save money, eat a quick lunch, and have more time for sightseeing.

- **Stay in a hotel room that has a mini-refrigerator.** Research hotels ahead of time and select one with this feature. Doing this enables you to refrigerate non-GMO dinner leftovers as well as perishable foods that you bring from home or purchase in natural food stores while traveling.

- **Research restaurants in the area you're going to visit.** Just as you scout restaurants in your hometown, you can do the same in different cities. If you're not sure about the availability of non-GMO, organic food at a particular eatery in your travel destination, call ahead and talk with the chef or manager. Get the addresses and phone numbers of the restaurants that sound best, map them, and print out driving instructions so you can easily find them—or use your smart phone to find this information. Special restaurants that serve delicious, non-GMO, organic and local food can make the difference between a trip and a real vacation.

- **Bring a restaurant translation food allergy card with you.** If you happen to travel to a foreign-speaking country, the chances are much better that you'll be avoiding most if not all of the GMOs found in North American food. Search online to learn the situation with GMOs in the country you'll be visiting. If you have allergies to GM foods such as corn and soy, download free gluten-free and allergy-free dining cards from GlutenFreePassport.com. They'll help you communicate with restaurant servers, chefs, and owners. *The food allergy cards include phrases to avoid the top common allergens, such as corn, dairy, egg, fish, gluten, peanuts, shellfish, soy, tree nuts and wheat, which of course include the most common GM offenders.* The cards are available in Dutch, French, German, Greek, Italian, Latvian, Portuguese, Russian, and Spanish.

Non-GMO Foods to Carry on Trips

The best foods to carry when you travel are those that are non-perishable, super nutritious, easy to transport, and of course non-GMO and gluten free. The following are some of the food items I most recommend to take on trips:

- **Non-GMO jerky**, such as Sophia's Survival Food mild beef jerky chews or Epic organic 100% grass-fed Lamb Bar. These products are free of GMOs, gluten, additives, and added sugars, and they come in handy, lightweight packages. The concentrated protein they contain provides slow-burning fuel that gives the body sustained energy to cope in difficult travel situations.

- **Cans of gluten-free tuna, salmon, or shrimp**, such as from those from Wild Planet Foods. These are best to take on road trips. Don't forget to pack a manual can opener.

- **Non-GMO protein bars**. Easy-to-transport, vegan sources of protein include SquareBar organic nutrition bars, Pure Food Bars, and Organic Food Bars.

- **Bags of non-GMO, gluten-free nuts or seeds**, such as Blue Diamond whole natural almonds, Eden Foods organic pumpkin seeds or pistachios, or Kaia Foods sprouted organic sunflower seeds. Nuts and seeds are packed with nutrients and they're hardy and easily transportable.

- **Nut or seed butter in handy packets.** They're ideal foods for providing a variety of nutrients, especially good fat to help satiate you, even if you eat only a spoonful. Look for single-serve squeeze packs of nut butter, such as organic almond butter, coconut butter, pecan butter, and macadamia butter, from Artisana.

- **Organic crackers**, such as Go Raw Flax Snax or Lydia's Organics Green Crackers or Ginger Nori Crackers. These grain-free crackers contain nutritious superfoods for much-needed nutrients to help fortify you during your travels.

- **Bags of fresh veggie sticks.** The more vegetables in the diet, the better it is for health, yet it's difficult to get enough vegetables while traveling. To balance out the protein you'll be eating, bring sturdy vegetable sticks for snacks.

- **Fresh fruit.** The best fruits for traveling—the hardiest, least apt to get bruised, most filling, and richest in digestion-regulating fiber—are apples. Some people carry bananas or peeled orange segments, but apples generally work best. Bring organic apples whenever possible.

- **Dried fruits or fruit bars.** Though not appropriate for my most sugar-sensitive clients, raisins, prunes, or other dried fruits are go-to sweet treats helpful for many people because they provide more nutrients and fiber than most sweets. They can be mixed and matched with nuts and seeds to make on-the-spot trail mixes. Other portable sweet "treats" include Non-GMO Project Verified That's It bars made with two kinds of fruit; widely available Larabars, made of dates, fruit, and nuts; and RBar products, which are similar but made with certified organic ingredients.

- **Water.** Water is a nutrient we need every day, but we sometimes get careless about drinking enough of it. Make sure to carry enough water with you on road trips, and buy a bottle and have it with you on plane rides to stay healthfully hydrated.

Now that you know the tricks of avoiding GMOs when you eat away from home, you can start building those skills in the outside world. Eating out non-GMO is hardest to do in the beginning and it can be rocky at times. However, the more you actively avoid GMOs away from home, the more you learn from newbie mistakes, and the more non-GMO coping skills in many different situations become second nature.

Chapter 13:

Educating Children and Teenagers about GMOs

Whether you're on the road or at home, avoiding genetically modified foods can be challenging on your own or with a partner. But it can be even more involved when you are raising young children or independent-minded teenagers. Young kids are heavily influenced by peer pressure, advertising, and marketing involving toys and games, and they may not be able to thoroughly understand the many compelling reasons to avoid GM foods, which look and taste exactly like real foods but are associated with many risks.

Most parents in America and Canada haven't learned enough to understand why and how their kids should avoid GM foods. But that's quickly changing. Many parents who learn that most GM foods are "pesticide plants" find that fact alone sufficiently motivating for them to avoid the main GMOs like corn and soy and choose more organic and Non-GMO Project Verified foods.

There also is a growing army of more adamant non-GMO parent activists who have put the pieces together about how much food has changed, how much sicker their children are than they were at the same age, and how other countries clearly label these ingredients or don't even allow them in their foods. As these parents educate their children, they become more involved in raising awareness in their community, talking to schools or churches, and taking other actions to help create a healthier food future for their children.

This chapter starts by explaining factors that motivate parents to influence children to avoid GMOs. Then it covers how children sometimes influence parents and how important it is for kids to be well informed so they can make intelligent food decisions on their own. It concludes by providing suggestions to help the whole family make changes toward healthier non-GMO food.

WHEN KIDS' ILLNESSES PROMPT PARENTS
TO LEARN ABOUT GMOS QUICKLY

When you're busy raising kids, maybe juggling a job as well, you may feel that it's hard enough to put food on the table, work within your budget, and get kids, especially little kids, to eat healthier foods. If you're like most overtaxed parents, you don't want to hear about how much our food has changed or that you unknowingly might have been feeding your children foods that look and taste the same as you ate but now have risky foreign ingredients in them. Learning that is emotionally painful, upsetting, and overwhelming.

If you feel that way, realize that you're not alone. Robyn O'Brien was a parent just like that, a busy married mother of four children. Though she is well educated, she was, in her own words, "completely disconnected and illiterate about what was in our food supply." All that changed quickly when her fourth child had a frightening allergic reaction at breakfast. O'Brien was plunged into the midst of a childhood epidemic she barely knew existed. She delved into understanding food allergy reactions and discovered the recent drastic changes to our food supply and dramatic increases in the rates of these health conditions in the last 20 years:[168]

- 400% increase in allergies

- 300% increase in asthma

- 400% increase in Attention Deficit Hyperactivity Disorder (ADHD)

- An increase of between 1,500 and 6,000% in the number of children with autism-spectrum disorders.

O'Brien began to realize that today's children are like canaries in the coal mine—if something is wrong in our food system, children, as a vulnerable, quickly developing segment of the population, are the first ones impacted. Although O'Brien felt she couldn't do everything about this monumental problem, she began making gradual changes in the foods she and her family ate. She also wrote about her discoveries in her book *The Unhealthy Truth* and founded AllergyKids, a foundation whose goal is to restore the health of our children and the integrity of our food supply.

Mother of three, Kathleen Hallal, had a similar experience. Although she herself had no allergies, her kids had 26 allergies between them! She realized something was very wrong with that situation. A few years ago, she went to a speech by farmer Howard Vlieger: The presentation visually showed pictures of how unhealthy animals were when they were fed herbicide-doused GM feed—and it all seemed to make sense. She learned more about GMOs on the Internet, talked with her husband, and switched her family to an organic diet, which helped improve all of her kids' health conditions.

As the cofounder of Moms Across America, a group designed to raise awareness and support mothers with solutions for eating GMO free, Hallal has found many other mothers who have had similar experiences. The group now has testimonials from more than 300 mothers who have seen improvements in autism, food and seasonal allergies, asthma, eczema, digestive issues, and autoimmune conditions after switching their kids to organic diets.

It's not well known as the national crisis that it is, but today's children are unhealthy, much sicker than their parents were as children. Besides the increase in allergies, asthma, ADHD, and autism-spectrum disorders, more than a third of children are now overweight or obese. Kids are being treated for high cholesterol and type 2 diabetes, which a few decades ago was called "adult-onset diabetes." There also have been runaway rates of pediatric cancer: There was a 55 percent increase from 1975 to 2005 in the incidence of leukemia in 0 to 14-year-olds and an 81 percent increase for acute lymphocytic leukemia, the most common type of leukemia.[169] The fact that so many children are so unwell lights a fire under many parents who never wanted to think much about food. Sometimes a parent may not necessarily want to make changes for herself but is willing to go to great lengths to make changes for her kids.

Generally speaking, women naturally gravitate at first to understanding the intimate relationship between food and health more than men, and as the primary caregivers of children, mothers tend to be the ones up all night trying to figure out what's going on with their kids. Husbands and fathers tend to be a bit more reluctant and questioning about going non-GMO and organic. But when they see stunning improvements in their children's (or their own) health conditions, they too become believers in the importance of eating non-GMO food—in other words, the incredible healing power of real, unadulterated food.

However, mothers make 85 percent of food purchases, so they're in the position to initiate the changes to non-GMO, organic food. The pace at which parents make changes is a matter of personal choice and judgment. Many mothers make gradual revisions in the family's diet, such as substituting or eliminating three or four items a week. However, when a child is very sick, mothers often swiftly make positive improvements in the foods they serve. This turns out to be a blessing in disguise because it quickly makes the whole family feel healthier. That's happening increasingly often.

WHEN PARENTS LEARN MORE GRADUALLY ABOUT GMOS

Some parents have kids who don't have (or don't appear to have) worrisome health conditions. One day out of the blue, those parents might see a segment about GMOs on the news or the Dr. Oz show. A while later, they might see a post on social media or hear friends talking about a variety of problems from GMOs, and troubling information about GMOs starts to sink in. The issue that catches their attention could be not wanting to have their children and themselves be guinea pigs in an experiment eating untested foods that might one day lead to health problems, wanting to avoid the pesticides that go hand in hand with most GMOs, or wanting to eat in a way that doesn't cause harm to our land or to bees, butterflies, and other wildlife.

Beginning Conversation About GMOs

The more parents learn, the more they want to explain to their children why they as a family are going to do their best to avoid eating genetically modified foods that sneakily look like real foods but aren't real foods on the inside. Each parent knows best how to approach her child and the approach might vary depending on the child's age. A beginning conversation with a young child might go something like this:

> "There have been changes in some common foods that weren't like that when I was your age, and I just recently became aware of those changes. Some plants that we eat today are made by scientists instead of nature."

> Your child might ask: Why do scientists make those plants and how do they do it?

> "They put genes from a different living thing into the cells of something we eat like corn. When scientists put those genes into corn, the corn doesn't die when you spray chemicals on it, or the corn might contain chemicals to kill bugs. It keeps the insects away and companies can use weed killers on it, but it probably isn't good for us or animals that eat it. That's why we want to do our best not to eat things that have been produced in this way."

> "Foods that are produced in this new way are called genetically modified, abbreviated as GMO. They're more like fake foods instead of real foods that Nature naturally provides."

Answer any questions your child has, then ask: "Will you please come to the grocery store with me and help me look for foods that aren't produced in this way? We can do it together, buy a lot of fresh vegetables and fruits, and look for packages that have a box with a butterfly on it (the non-GMO symbol) or a circle that says USDA Organic."

It's best not to make the first conversation too long. Explain the subject to kids in bits and pieces so they can slowly digest the information, just as you likely learned it. Then let them research it on their own by reading kid-friendly information on the Internet. They may come back to you with questions, and you can gradually give them more information.

Be sure to make a copy of the Word Game in Appendix B and let them see how many names of genetically modified foods they can find. Trust me when I say: Kids get totally engaged in and love playing that Word Game!

When Children Learn About GMOs First

An exciting development in the non-GMO movement is that children sometimes learn about genetically modified foods before their parents do, then they convince the whole family to change their habits to avoid GM foods! After learning on their own and talking with their family, some of these children spread the word to peers their own age and go on to become public speakers and agents of change.

That's exactly what happened with Birke Baehr who, at age 8, began researching about our industrial food system and learned about GMOs. He put some information together and talked with family members and then friends about what he was learning on the Internet.

In 2010, at age 11, Birke gave a five-minute TEDx talk entitled "What's Wrong with Our Food System" that went viral on YouTube with more than 2 million total views. Two years later, Birke wrote a picture book entitled *Birke on the Farm: A Boy's Search for Real Food*. It tells the story of his journey of discovery about food and farming and is designed to help small children learn about the food system, including GMOs. To learn more, visit BirkeOnTheFarm.com.

Birke is 15 years old now. He has become an internationally known speaker and youth advocate for sustainable food and agriculture and is passionate about continuing to spread his message of change in our food system, as he says, "one kid at a time."

I began to look into this stuff on the Internet, in books, in documentary films, in my travels with my family. I discovered the dark side of the industrialized food system.

First, there's genetically engineered seeds and organisms. That is when a seed is manipulated in a laboratory to do something not intended by nature. Like taking the DNA of a fish and putting it into the DNA of a tomato.

YUCK! Don't get me wrong: I like fish and tomatoes, but this is just creepy!

...Some people say organic or local is more expensive. But is it really? With all the things I've been learning about the food system, it seems to me that we can either pay the farmer or the hospital.

> — Birke Baehr, at age 11, at a 2010 TEDx talk in Asheville, NC

It's important for everyone to know about GMOs and especially kids because this issue with GMOs is not only impacting our future, it's impacting us today. People are unknowingly eating GMOs and it could be making them sick and severely damaging our ecosystem at the same time.

— Rachel Parent, a 15-year-old Canadian non-GMO advocate, speaker, and founder of Kids Right to Know

MORE YOUTH ACTIVISTS

Another dedicated non-GMO youth activist today is Rachel Parent from Canada. She learned about GMOs at 11 years old when she was trying to decide what to speak on for a school project. Rachel discovered that GMOs not only impacted our health but also the environment, and she knew she had to speak about the topic. She talked with her family about what she learned and, as a family, they decided to change the food in their cabinets. "As soon as we did this, my respiratory allergies and digestive and skin disorders went away and I became a healthy kid again," she wrote in an email interview with me.

In August 2013, Rachel became an Internet sensation for her cool-headed debate about GMOs against Kevin O'Leary, co-host of *The Lang & O'Leary Exchange* show on Canadian television. The YouTube video of it has been viewed close to 3 million times.

She is a self-motivated 15-year-old who has traveled to Brazil's Amazon to witness forest devastation brought about from planting genetically modified soy. She also founded Kids Right to Know (KidsRightToKnow. com) and speaks throughout Canada. Plus, she has publicly asked for a meeting with Canada's Minister of Health Rona Ambrose to have an open discussion about food safety and share peer-reviewed scientific research about the dangers of genetically engineered food. Via her website and YouTube videos, she is enlisting the help of the Canadian public to push for that meeting.

Birke Baehr and Rachel Parent may be the most well-known non-GMO youth advocates but they are not by any means the only ones. Some children learn about GMOs from their parents, then they get great ideas to try to evoke changes in business by large organizations and further public awareness of the issue.

In 2013, 6-year-old Alicia Serratos from Orange County, California, who already knew about GMOs, was one such little girl. She discovered that Girl Scout cookies contained GMOs and asked her mother why the cookies could not be reformulated with non-GMO ingredients. Alicia and her mother talked about it and decided to create a Change.org online petition entitled "Girl Scouts: Please make cookies without GMOs." The petition had close to 30,000 signatures as of July 4, 2014. Underneath the petition is a post with a link to download a kid-friendly coloring book that Alicia made by hand to help kids learn about GMOs.

EDUCATING CHILDREN, NOT DEPRIVING THEM

The children are our future. We've all heard that popular saying. What is instilled in the youth today—thoughts, beliefs, and teachings—will greatly affect the way the world turns out. What will our future be like if we shield children and keep them uneducated about GMOs? Let's face it: That kind of future would not be a pretty picture. We simply can't afford to keep kids uneducated about food.

Mother and freelance writer Christina Le Beau has developed a website and blog called Spoonfed (Spoonfedblog.net), which is completely devoted to topics surrounding her website's tagline, "raising kids to think about the food they eat." What follows are a few thoughts directly from her website:[170] [171]

> Amid rampant food-industry manipulation and misinformation, our best hope for raising healthy children is to raise food-literate children—kids who think critically, challenge the status quo and make smart choices even when we can't choose for them.
>
> I want people to rethink their assumptions about kids and food...
>
> Kids are... smart. Scary smart. Smart enough to understand how food choices affect their bodies and the environment. It's not enough to feed our kids real, healthful food. We need to teach them *why* we're doing it. Children need tools to make good choices even after we stop filling their plates. And they need parents and other advocates to speak out against a prevailing but deeply flawed food culture that spoonfeeds kids and hopes we won't notice.

I completely agree. Remember it's not just GMOs that are a big problem. It's sugar, refined flour, refined oils, food additives, pesticides, and all the other ingredients I talked about in Chapter 8 that are making both adults and children sick. Our food system is in crisis, and children need to be brought into the conversation in a way that encourages critical thinking to make well-informed decisions so they can play their part in helping to create the healthy food system we need.

Another important point Le Beau raises is that educating kids is not about depriving them in a draconian way. Kids *can* indulge in childhood pleasures, but even party meals and treats should be made of higher-quality ingredients than the fake food ingredients normally served in typical foods to children.[172] You can give children non-GMO Halloween candy, candy canes during the holidays, birthday cakes, and more. Just do it *on occasion* instead of allowing your children regular, constant hits of sugar day in and day out. When you give them higher-quality real foods, children often immediately notice a difference in how much better the foods taste and how much better they feel than they did when they ate junkier alternatives. That gives them the information and positive experience they need to motivate them to choose healthier food options in the future. (When people are in touch with the connection between what they eat and how they feel, neither kids nor adults want to consciously choose foods that make them sick!)

TIPS FOR GOING NON-GMO AS A FAMILY

No matter whether a parent or child learns about genetically engineered foods first, making changes in longstanding eating habits always works best when everybody in the family is involved. Making those changes also has to begin at home where we have the most control.

Just as individuals have to start somewhere and slowly improve their diet from where they begin, so too do families. You know all the individuals in your family, so trust your judgment and weigh emotional and social considerations. If you buy and cook most of the foods in your home, begin taking action against GMOs to the degree you deem best. You can be stricter or less strict later on, but the most important thing is to start somewhere.

General Guidelines for Inside The Home

Begin by getting problematic GMOs out of the house (either slowly or all at once), and bring in healthier alternatives. This means avoiding processed foods and eating more whole foods (i.e., fresh fruits, vegetables, nuts, seeds, and clean meats).

Keep in mind that there are organic alternatives to every kind of food. If your family doesn't feel like it can give up certain foods—tacos, for example—make sure to buy organic, non-GMO ingredients to prepare them. As time goes on, gradually emphasize more vegetables in place of grain-based foods like taco shells. Try taco salads instead for better health. Also, transition to using grass-fed meats in family favorites such as hamburgers, meatballs, and meatloaf. By using non-GMO and organic food substitutions, you can make any food that your family likes non-GMO.

The more you can encourage family members to be engaged in the change to non-GMO foods, the better the process typically goes. See if you can motivate everyone in the household to follow the month-long series of tips in the Eat GMO-Free Challenge in Chapter 7 to learn how to eat real food again. Get kids involved by playing the word game, going shopping with you, cooking with you, and gardening with you. Ask your children to choose new non-GMO, organic foods or recipes the whole family can try. The more that kids are connected with where their food comes from, the less likely they will want to consciously eat GM foods. Plus, when kids learn from their parents how to cook simple, healthy foods, they gain a skill that will benefit them their entire lives.

I understand that the transition to non-GMO food doesn't always go smoothly with no bumps. Everything I wrote in Chapter 5—that changing longstanding habits is an up-and-down process and we all make mistakes—applies to families, too. Be sure to deal with your and other family members' feelings, find support (from online resources in the Resources section), and be patient with the process. When you get GM products out of your house, you know for sure that your children won't be eating these foods at home—and this is a big part of keeping them (and all other members of the family) well.

General Guidelines for Outside The Home

When your child is away from home, it's much more difficult to control what he eats. That's why it's so important to educate your child about the many reasons to avoid GMOs and other fake food ingredients, so he can make good decisions on his own.

To help your child eat healthy foods when he's away from home, try these tips:

- **Plan ahead.** This was emphasized in Chapter 5, but it bears repeating. Parents need to look at outside events that are coming up on the schedules of each child and family member and get prepared.

- **Always pack lunch.** This is the best way to help your child avoid the GMOs that are in most school lunches.

- **Bring non-GMO snacks for the family when you go to the movies.** If a child is going to go to a movie theater with a friend, encourage him to pack healthy snacks, such as non-GMO popcorn, nuts, or kale chips.

If you help your child eat a nutritious, low-sugar, whole-food diet at home and educate him about the reasons why, you have laid the groundwork for good health. When you do that, it may not be such a bad thing for your child to have a few foods that he doesn't normally eat when he's out with his friends. He'll likely notice how much worse he feels after eating those junky foods and be less apt to eat them the next time he's out on his own.

However, if your child comes back from camp or a long day out with a friend eating unhealthy foods and experiences a dramatic increase in allergy and asthma symptoms or other health issues, gently point out that you see a connection between when he eats fake foods, including GMOs, and when he experiences troublesome health reactions. Emphasize the idea that it doesn't matter what everyone else eats—it matters what foods are good or not good for *him*. Be sure to reassure him that his true friends will still like him even if he doesn't always eat what they eat, and reinforce his self-esteem. To make eating non-GMO easier for your child socially speaking, give him tasty, non-GMO and organic snack foods and occasional sweets to share with his friends.

Parenting teenagers can be extra challenging. In the naturally rebellious stage they're in, teenagers may sometimes eat junky foods with abandon, which means GMOs galore. Although it's frustrating that you can't control everything your teenage children eat and do, you must make them understand that they are responsible for the health consequences of their actions—whether that means more skin breakouts, more digestive issues, more weight gain, more allergy symptoms, or any other possible adverse health effects.

Over time, they generally learn what's best for them. As one mother whose children have autoimmune conditions said to me, "For a while, it was a big challenge trying to encourage them to avoid both GMOs and their food allergens, and it took a lot of time and trial and error. But eventually they made the connection and got sick and tired of being sick and tired from what they ate."

General Guidelines for Special Occasions

With so many special occasions for families to celebrate in life — birthdays, graduations, anniversaries, major accomplishments, and holidays—it's important to be creative making those gatherings fun and festive without including foods that contain unhealthy GMOs. To accomplish this goal, you might let other dietary standards slide just a bit for a day. But, often, you don't have to compromise. Try making the Simple Delicious Cake for a child's birthday party and don't tell anyone it's GMO free (as well as gluten free and dairy free). I bet your party guests will never know the difference and might even comment on how tasty the cake is.

Kids tend to like finger food, party food on toothpicks and food in which a fun process is involved preparing it. Try allowing children to choose their own toppings for tacos (this works if your child can tolerate corn) or letting them top gluten-free, non-GMO pizza crust with the ingredients of their choice. For party desserts, a low-sugar option that kids usually love is berries or other pieces of fruit on toothpicks with homemade whipped cream or coconut milk cream to dip their fruit in.

Another good strategy is to ask your child to choose whatever he wants—his favorite non-GMO food—for his party. Special occasions are meant for sharing good times and celebrating life, and eating non-GMO, organic, real food is the best, most proactive celebration of life I can think of.

Chapter 14:

Other Ways to Take Action Against GMOs

The focus of this book is to provide information on how to avoid GM foods so we can use our consumer power efficiently. When enough of us understand and put into action the nitty-gritty details of how to avoid GMOs in the foods we purchase, companies will stop using them. For that reason, writing this consumer-oriented book is how I felt I could best contribute to the non-GMO movement.

People with other talents and interests are taking different actions, all of which play a part in creating a fast-growing movement of consumer awareness and rejection of GMOs. Although it's not necessary to do anything more than be a non-GMO shopper as much as you can possibly be, if you feel the need to become more involved to help to eradicate GMOs, there are plenty of ways to contribute. The following is not a complete list, but it's a rundown of some main alternative (but still complementary) ways to take action against GMOs.

GRASSROOTS EFFORTS FOR GMO BANS

Given that GM foods have been unlabeled and basically unregulated for nearly two decades in the United States and Canada, growing numbers of people are deciding to put their efforts toward a combination of GMO boycotts and bans. In other words, they are using their purchasing power to let companies know it's a liability to have GMOs in food products, and they're also working toward passing local bans that prevent genetically modified crops from being planted, like those that have taken place in other regions and countries. To learn how to ban GMOs in your city or county, visit InternationalGMOBanAlliance.org.

If you need to be convinced about bans, consider that during the past 20 years that GM foods have been unlabeled in our marketplace, GMOs have continued to spread through wind drift and have contaminated more and more conventional and organic crops. Because this type of contamination is unique to GM crops grown out in the open environment, farmers are leading the push to convince people to work toward bans. Barbara H. Peterson writes convincingly on FarmsWars.Info about how frustrating it is to be a farmer trying to find alfalfa for animal feed that is not contaminated with GMOs and how GM crops are doing terrible harm to we the people and our planet.

In a video on her post "Monsanto is Not 'Too Big to Fail,'" Peterson says:[173]

> If labeling is the first priority, then by the time we get around to banning (GMOs), contamination will be so rampant that there will be nothing left that doesn't require labeling.
>
> And we know that labeling is routinely manipulated and the exemptions so huge that a GMO elephant could walk through them. Meanwhile, (GMOs) continue to be grown and the contamination continues.
>
> And what will happen when the threshold for GMO-free isn't really *GMO-free*? Then the labelists will simply raise the threshold of acceptable contamination so that the words really don't mean what they say anymore. And "GMO-free" will actually mean 90% GMO-free, or 80%, or whatever bar they choose to raise the level to, to accommodate the level of acceptable contamination that we are being conditioned to accept.

According to investigative reporter Jon Rappoport, labeling initiatives seem to solve the problem of GMOs, but they barely scratch the surface of it. The initiatives are what he calls "soft," and they misdirect attention, reduce the much-needed outrage against genetically modified seed companies such as Monsanto, and suck up money and volunteers that could otherwise be working toward campaigns for bans either locally in their community or nationally.

In "Are GMO Ballot Measures Just Another Covert Op?" Rappoport writes:[174]

> …Monsanto can deal with GMO labeling wherever it's passed.
>
> The real threat to Monsanto is a massive popular uprising against the corporation and its horrendous desecration of food. For example, when a U.S. county passes a law against the growing of any GMO crop within its borders, that's a dagger.
>
> Were such a movement to spread, Monsanto would be shaking in its boots.

For these and other reasons I explain in Appendix G, I favor GMO bans over labeling. Some people say we have to settle for labeling because countywide bans can't be accomplished. However, we know that's not true. Just read the many examples below of counties that have passed bans against GMOs, particularly in the last few years:

- In 2004, Mendocino and Marin counties in California became the first counties in the United States to pass GMO bans.

- In 2012, Washington Initiative Measure No. 2012-4 passed, which makes it illegal to "propagate, cultivate, raise or grow plants, animals and other organisms which have been genetically modified" in San Juan County, Washington.[175]

- In 2013, the Kauai County Council enacted Ordinance 960, the first local law in the United States that specifically regulates the cultivation of existing GMO crops. In addition, the mayor of the Big Island of Hawaii signed a bill into law that bans all future plantings of GMOs and prohibits biotech companies from operating on the Big Island.[176] [177]

- Also, in 2013, two city councilmen proposed a motion to make the city of Los Angeles a GMO-Free zone, the largest one in the country, by banning the growth, sale and distribution of GM seeds and plants anywhere in the city.[178]

- In 2014, residents in both Jackson and Josephine counties in Oregon passed bans on planting GM crops.[179]

- In November 2014, a temporary ban on genetically modified crops will be voted on by the residents in Hawaii's Maui County, which is made up of Maui, Molokai and Lanai—and an ordinance prohibiting the cultivation and growing of GMOs will be voted on by residents in Humboldt County, California.[180] [181]

GRASSROOTS EFFORTS FOR GMO LABELING

If you feel drawn to labeling efforts, there are many ways to take part. My view is: Why fight for labeling, which takes a long time to achieve and is likely to be a false security blanket, when we can become savvy consumers and avoid GM foods right now? The only reason I can think of is to raise consumer awareness about the problems with GMOs. If that's your reason, I completely respect that.

The history of other types of labeling unfortunately shows us that when federal labeling occurs, compromises are made. The standards end up favoring industry over people's health, and there is a lack of monitoring and policing of companies that don't adhere to the law. The foods sometimes are not completely free of the offending ingredient that people are trying to avoid (such as what happened with "gluten free"); there can be exemptions (such as milk, meat, restaurant items, and alcohol being exempt from most proposed GMO labeling laws); or kids have allergic reactions to food allergens that aren't supposed to be in the labeled foods (as has occurred with "allergen-free" labeling). Virtually nothing is done to companies that mislabel their products. (Again, read Appendix G for more information.)

I think it's a mistake to naïvely believe that that the government, especially the FDA, is protecting us or will protect us if a labeling law is passed. This is the same FDA that allowed GM foods unlabeled in the market in the first place. The situation with GMOs is so urgent, we have to take the power into our hands now: Use the step-by-step instructions of how to avoid GM foods detailed in this book and help create a tipping point of consumer rejection against GM foods, no matter what happens with labeling.

GRASSROOTS ACTIVISM AND POLITICAL ACTION

Do you feel a need to help in the activism and political action arena? There's plenty of need for that. As labeling and banning efforts have kicked into higher gear, many frustrating, maddening developments slanted toward corporate control and favoritism over the will of the people have occurred. In early 2013, there was the Farmer Assurance Provision, more colloquially known as the "Monsanto Protection Act," which caused such outrage and protest that it fortunately was eventually allowed to expire. In 2014, a bill (HR 4432), which has been called the "Denying Americans the Right-to-Know Act" (DARK Act), was introduced in the U.S. Congress: It would prevent states from enacting laws requiring mandatory labeling of GMOs.

Perhaps even more disconcerting, over the past year or two, secret trade agreements known as the Trans-Pacific Partnership (TPP) and Trans-Atlantic Free Trade Agreement (TAFTA) have been being negotiated behind closed doors by corporate interests. According to the non-profit organization Food & Water Watch, a provision inside the TPP will allow companies to challenge—as illegal trade barriers—any government policies that purportedly infringe on corporate profits. In short, a corporation could sue federal, state and local governments if it believes that a law or regulation will negatively impact its bottom line. This is scary in all sorts of ways.[182]

"Many people don't know that these secret negotiations may undermine efforts on both sides of the Atlantic to protect our food, our health, and our environment," said Debbie Barker, International Program Director at the Center for Food Safety in a press release. "Those of us concerned about the food we feed our families must get involved before it is too late."[183]

Because of these outrageously undemocratic developments by any standards, more people who never considered themselves activists have realized that democracy is not a spectator sport. They've joined a number of national non-GMO and food safety groups to become more informed about what elected officials and lobbyists are doing to block grassroots efforts to protect food safety, and they call and write elected officials to vote against bills that favor corporate interests over public welfare.

If you want to play a part in a collective movement to protect our food, consider joining the email lists of non-profit groups, such as the Center for Food Safety, the Organic Consumers Association, Food Democracy Now, and many others that are leading grassroots food safety activism efforts. The political climate is such these days that many say we can't just shop our way to more democratic control over our food. We have to hold more elected officials accountable for how they vote on various bills, let them know we are watching what they are doing, and ultimately elect representatives and senators who align with what we want. The only way to effectively do that is to receive regular news updates and action alerts from organizations that specialize in protecting our food rights.

TARGETED BOYCOTT, PETITION, OR CALLING CAMPAIGNS

You can also get involved in targeted boycotts, petitions, or calling campaigns against certain companies or to certain organizations. Diana Reeves, a mother who was completely discouraged after she put an incredible amount of time and effort into labeling legislation in Connecticut that failed, decided there had to be a better way to change the system. She started GMO Free USA, which now has 350,000 followers on Facebook, to collectively speak to and force large food manufacturers to come clean with the ingredients they use in their products. "If they won't remove GMOs, we will boycott them until they do," she says.

GMO Free USA's first campaign began with boycotting the Kellogg Company, which heavily markets to children and sells the same products abroad *without* using genetically engineered ingredients, but sells GMO-containing products here in the United States! GMO Free USA also now has boycotts against Nestle's Gerber, which does not use GMOs in its baby foods in Europe, and against Girl Scout Cookies. GMO Free Canada is a sister organization that often works in concert with GMO Free USA. You can learn more on their Facebook pages.

Other groups that coordinate targeted campaigns that you might be interested in include:

- Moms Across America (MomsAcrossAmerica.com), which is petitioning the Centers for Disease Control and the Food and Drug Administration to conduct testing on GM foods and glyphosate (Roundup herbicide), and which also has coordinated marches the past few years to raise awareness about GMOs in July 4th parades across the country.

- FoodBabe.com (food watchdog Vani Hari) who investigates harmful ingredients in many foods and solicits an army of followers to pressure food companies and restaurants to remove those ingredients.

- GMO Inside (GMOInside.org), which has campaigns against top infant formula companies Similac, Enfamil, and Gerber; Honey Nut Cheerios; Chobani yogurt; Dean Foods, which is one of the largest processors and direct distributors of dairy products; and against Starbucks to serve only organic (non-GMO) milk in its beverages.

FINANCIAL ACTION

A completely different way to take action against the stacked-in-favor-of-corporations situation with GMOs is to ditch mutual funds that own large volumes of stock from the major biotech companies. In Chapter 1, I explained about the current Operation Monsanto Stock Plunge campaign, which is encouraging people to sell Fidelity, Vanguard and State Street mutual funds that own and control enormous volumes of Monsanto stock.

Since the campaign launched in the spring of 2014, thousands of Americans concerned about what they're eating—and what their investments are funding in the way of risky GMOs—have been calling their financial advisors and discovering that they inadvertently own shares of Monsanto's stock that were hiding in their mutual funds, 401K, or pension funds. They in turn have asked their advisors to sell those funds and invest in more socially and environmentally responsible ones. Given that making money is the primary concern of corporations, financial action may be one of the most effective types of action. You can learn more about this effort at FoodDemocracyNow.org.

GROWING YOUR OWN FOOD

Here's a more earthy way to take action: Grow your own food from non-GMO organic or heirloom seeds. For some people, that might mean growing herbs in pots in a small apartment in the city. For others, that might mean having their own land, or plots in community gardens, and growing a variety of fresh produce. Some even raise chickens on non-GMO feed to have their own sources of freshly laid eggs.

If you enjoy gardening, it's good exercise, and it puts you in touch with the seasonal availability of foods. Most say growing fresh produce is rewarding, the produce is more nutritious, and eating it tastes much better than the produce offered in supermarkets. Growing your own food or purchasing from farms in your area helps build a stronger community-oriented agricultural system, which food experts agree is necessary to create a sustainable alternative to our current large-scale industrial food system.

SEED SAVING

Another important part of the non-GMO movement is not just growing food from heirloom or historical seeds, but saving those seeds and passing them onto others as farmers have traditionally done. It's hard to believe that in the past century, 90 percent of our seed varieties of vegetables have gone extinct! More and more people are realizing that we need to protect the right to use historical seeds—or lose that right. Toward that goal, the Open Source Seed Initiative was launched in the spring of 2014 to provide an alternative to the patent-protected seeds sold by major producers such as Monsanto and DuPont that generally prohibit farmers from planting those seeds the following year. The Open Source Seed project aims to provide a way to free both the farmer and the seed for a future where plant genetic resources may remain unrestricted.

Seed saving and open-source seed exchanging are vital for protecting the future of our food. If you are interested in getting involved in this way, learn more by watching the documentary *Open Sesame: The Story of Seeds* (OpenSesameMovie.com) and visit OpenSourceSeedInitiative. org for more info.

COMMUNITY INVOLVEMENT AND EDUCATION

If you have a desire to help raise awareness and educate fellow citizens in your community, consider joining the Institute for Responsible Technology's Tipping Point Network at ResponsibleTechnology.org. The network coordinator can put you in touch with a non-GMO group in your area, and you can decide which ways you can contribute that are fun and easy for you. Your contributions could be as simple as spreading the word on Facebook or talking to people at your school or church. Or they could be more involved such as planning and organizing large community-wide movie showings, presentations, and legislation or banning efforts. The latter can be a lot of work at times, but networking with others is a great deal of fun and much more effective at bringing positive change in your community.

DONATIONS

If you find a 501(c)(3) tax-exempt non-profit group that is doing good work you believe in, consider giving it a financial contribution. A small non-profit organization that is fighting against moneyed corporate interests always has things it wants to do but can't because of lack of finances. When you give a donation, it just might be enough to allow the organization to hire more staff or purchase supplies and resources it needs to complete large-scale education and action campaigns.

SOME FINAL WORDS

The fight for non-GMO, organic food is a numbers game: There are a lot more of us consumers who don't want GM foods in our food supply than there are biotech companies who are fighting to keep them in. It's just a matter of time before our numbers and efforts win out. If each of us spreads the word and contributes in ways that resonate with our interests and talents, even if that's just to shop non-GMO and let a few others know the truth about GM foods, getting these inconceivable, dangerous, corporate-created pseudo-foods out of our food supply is going to happen sooner rather than later.

What I wrote at the end of Chapter 4 bears repeating: With the vision of a healthy, organic, locally centered food system firmly in our hearts and minds, we can create the change in our food system that we seek.

Mahatma Gandhi famously said: "Be the change you wish to see in the world." It's now time to be that change.

SECTION 3:

Additional Helpful Information

Appendix A:
List of Hidden GMO Ingredients

When listed as a food additive, the following are most probably from GMO sources:

Artificial Sweetener
Aspartame:
    AminoSweet
    NutraSweet
    Equal
    Canderel
    BeneVia
    E951
Baking Powder
Brown Sugar
Canola Oil
Caramel Color
Cellulose
Citric Acid
Cobalamin (Vitamin B12)
Colorose
Condensed Milk
Confectioners Sugar
Corn Flour
Corn Masa
Corn Meal
Corn Oil
Corn Sugar
Corn Syrup
Cornstarch

Cottonseed Oil
Cyclodextrin
Cystein
Dextrin
Dextrose
Diacetyl
Glutamate
Glutamic Acid
Glycerin
Glycerol Monooleate
Glycine
Hemicellulose
High-Fructose Corn Syrup
Hydrogenated Starch
Hydrolyzed Vegetable Protein
Inositol
Inverse Syrup
Invert Sugar
Inversol
Isoflavones
Lactic Acid
Lecithin
Leucine
Lysine
Maliltol

Malt

Malt Syrup

Malt Extract

Maltodextrin

Maltose

Mannitol

Methylcellulose

Milk Powder

Milo Starch

Modified Food Starch

Mono and diglycerides

Monosodium Glutamate (MSG)

Nutrasweet

Oleic Acid

Phenylalanine

Protein Isolate

Rapeseed oil

Shoyu

Sorbitol

Soy Flour

Soy Isolates

Soy Lecithin

Soy Milk

Soy Oil

Soy Protein

Soy Protein Isolate

Soy Sauce

Starch

Stearic Acid

Sugar (not cane sugar)

Tamari

Tempeh

Teriyaki

Textured Vegetable Protein

Threonine

Tocopherols (Vitamin E)

Tofu

Trehalose

Triglyceride

Vegetable Fat

Vegetable Oil

Vitamin B12

Vitamin E

Whey

Whey Powder

Xanthan Gum

Xylitol (from corn)

Adapted with permission from the Institute for Responsible Technology

Appendix B:
Find the GM Foods Word Game

For Kids and Adults

See how many foods and drinks you can find that are common sources
of genetically modified ingredients. When you eat non-GMO, these
items should be avoided (unless they are organic or non-GMO) to
protect your health and the planet's health.

*Hint: Words will be spelled across and up and down,
not spelled backwards.*

```
W H A T A R E W E E A T I N G F R A N K E N F O O D S
C O R N C H I P S V O A S O F T D R I N K S P M P O O
O L G A O I S T O X I C A N D U N H E A L T H Y T R D
L I N P R C A N D Y M O V E P T Y U C K Y S T U F F A
A B D G N M O S T C O O K I E S R I S K Y Z O N S H P
U N L A B E L E D A N D U N T E S T E D X T C U T S O
E N V I R O N M E N T A L L Y U N F R I E N D L Y U P
G R S W E E T S C A N O L A O I L I S G M O G M O G M
A N I M A L S A V O I D T H E M L A B R A T S T T A N
R E A L D A N G E R M A N Y C E R E A L S T O F U R D
S O Y M I L K U N S A F E S A Y N O T O G M O S B Y E
```

Courtesy of *Going Against GMOs* by Melissa Diane Smith
www.goingagainstgmos.com - www.melissadianesmith.com
Feel free to copy and distribute this page for education purposes.

Answers To Word Game

There are 13 to 17 answers depending on how you name the foods.

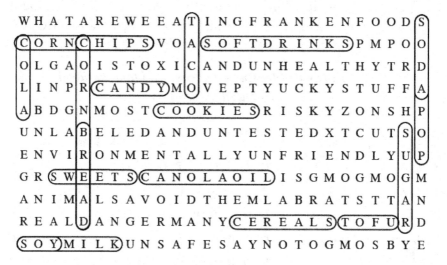

Appendix C:
Test Your GMO Knowledge Quiz

Take this quiz and test your knowledge about GMOs, then pass the test onto others to raise awareness about this timely topic.

Test Your Knowledge

1. True or False: An easy way to remember the five major genetically modified crops in our food supply is to remember that they all begin with the letter "c".

2. True or False: The two main traits given to foods that are genetically modified are to produce their own insecticide or to be resistant to herbicides that kill other plants.

3. True or False: The terms "genetically modified" and "genetically engineered" mean different things.

4. True or False: In the genetic modification process, biotech scientists often use viruses and bacteria to invade cells of plants and insert foreign genes.

5. True or False: The only sweeteners likely to contain genetically modified organisms (GMOs) on the market are those made from corn—i.e., corn syrup, high-fructose corn syrup, and fructose.

6. True or False: No cases of illness have ever been reported by people who have eaten foods that have been genetically modified or ingested products in which GMOs were used.

7. True or False: One of the main corporations involved in making and patenting genetically modified seeds is a top chemical company that manufactured the chemicals Agent Orange and DDT.

8. True or False: Polls conducted by the three major TV networks show that most Americans want genetically modified foods labeled.

9. True or False: Animal studies indicate that there are only two health risks associated with eating GM foods: infertility and reproductive problems.

10. True or False: Genetically modified *E. coli* bacteria is used in the production of recombinant bovine growth hormone (rBGH), which is injected into some cows to boost milk production.

11. True or False: One way to identify GM produce in the grocery store is to look for a label on the produce item with a 5-digit PLU code starting with the number 8.

Quiz courtesy of *Going Against GMOs* by Melissa Diane Smith.
Feel free to copy and distribute this page for education purposes.

Answers to the Quiz:

1. **False.** Three of the five—corn, canola, and cottonseed—begin with the letter "c". The other two begin with "s". They are soy and sugar from sugar beets.

2. **True.** The five most common GM foods are genetically modified to either produce their own insecticide or to tolerate herbicides that kill other plants—or both.

3. **False.** "Genetically modified" and "genetically engineered" mean the same thing—altering genes or inserting genes from one living organism into another—and the two terms are used interchangeably.

4. **True.** Viruses and bacteria have the ability to invade cells, so one of the key ways biotech scientists overcome the natural barriers that genes have against genetic material from another species is by using some type of bacteria or virus that is carrying foreign genetic material to penetrate the host cell.

5. **False.** Sweeteners made from corn, more than 80 percent of which is genetically modified, are likely to contain GMOs. But so is sugar, which is usually a combination of sugar from sugar cane and sugar from GM sugar beets. Also, the artificial sweetener aspartame, found in Nutrasweet and Equal, is a genetically modified product.

6. **False.** In 2000, reports came in to environmental groups and the Food and Drug Administration from people who said they got sick or suffered severe allergic reactions after eating taco shells made from a type of genetically modified corn called StarLink that was not approved for human consumption; that was before nationwide recalls of the products were issued. In 1989, more than a thousand people became ill or disabled and about 100 Americans died after taking L-tryptophan supplements from one company that used genetically engineered bacteria in the production of the product. According to some American Academy of Environmental Medicine physicians, patients are probably seeing negative health effects right now from

eating GM foods but they or their doctors don't realize that GM foods may be contributing to those health conditions.

7. **True.** Monsanto, the biggest seller of GM crop seeds in the world, is a top chemical company that manufactured DDT and Agent Orange. It is the producer of the leading weed killer Roundup and most of the GM seeds the corporation produces are genetically engineered to be "Roundup Ready"—in other words, to withstand applications of Roundup that kills other plants.

8. **True.** A 2001 ABC News poll found that 93 percent of people think the government should require mandatory labeling of GM foods. In 2011, a CBS/*New York Times* blog poll found that 83 percent of U.S. consumers are bothered by the presence of GMOs in food and 89 percent want GM foods labeled. A 2011 MSNBC poll found that 96 percent want GM foods labeled.

9. **False.** Based on animal research, infertility and reproductive problems are two serious health risks associated with eating GM foods, but there are numerous others, including immune system problems, accelerated aging, disruption of insulin and cholesterol regulation, gastrointestinal problems, and organ damage, according to the American Academy of Environmental Medicine.

10. **True.** The United States is one of only a few nations that allows the use of genetically modified rBGH in dairy cattle. However, in recent years, consumer reaction and concerns in the U.S. have prompted Wal-Mart, Starbucks, and many dairies to either not use or to stop using rBGH. Some dairies still do, though. To avoid it, look for milk products labeled USDA Organic or rBGH-free or rBST-free.

11. **False.** That's an urban legend that's circulated far and wide, but it's a misconception. Looking for a 5-digit PLU code that starts with 8 isn't helpful for identifying GM produce items because many companies don't want consumers to know which foods are GMO, so no company uses a number starting with 8, says leading non-GMO

advocate Jeffrey Smith. To steer clear of GM produce, know that the only fruits and vegetables at this point that may be genetically modified are papaya (from Hawaii and China), and some zucchini, yellow squash, and corn on the cob. Avoid these produce items or seek out organic forms or those that boast a non-GMO sign.

Appendix D:
How Good Is Your Food Shopping Savvy?

Take this questionnaire to see what you know and what you don't to make more informed decisions when you shop.

Natural, organic, gluten-free, free-range, grass-fed, and more. There are so many different terms and so many different ways to read labels, it's a lot for shoppers to sort through, grasp, and comprehend! Many marketing terms are confusing, and let's face it: Some are downright misleading. As a nutrition counselor, I find that most consumers don't know exactly what various terms mean but have ideas of what they think they mean—ideas that are often wrong. Misunderstanding terms on labels causes many of us shoppers to sometimes, maybe far more often than we realize, purchase products we don't really want to.

To buy the kind of food you really want, it's important to become educated and super savvy as a consumer. Take the questionnaire below that I developed to test your knowledge. After you answer the questions, view the answers to get the real scoop on what various food label terms mean and what the FDA and food laws require, and get up to date on any information you may not have known before.

Test Your Consumer Savvy

Avoiding Gluten and Food Allergens

1. True or False: "Gluten free" on a label means the product is completely free of the problematic protein gluten.

2. True or False: Food manufacturers are required to identify on food labels when any of the top eight food allergens are in the ingredients of a product and also when food allergens might be present in the manufacturing facility.

3. True or False: The top eight food allergens that are required to be identified on food labels are wheat, soy, milk, peanuts, tree nuts, fish, shellfish and eggs.

Choosing Natural and Organic Foods

4. True or False: Buying foods that are labeled "Natural" is a good way to avoid foods that contain laboratory created genetically modified organisms (GMOs).

5. True or False: Food that is labeled USDA Organic is produced without using GMOs, ionizing radiation, most conventional pesticides, and fertilizers made with synthetic ingredients or sewage sludge.

Understanding Free-Range and Grass-Fed

6. True or False: Chicken and eggs labeled "free range" means they are from chickens that freely forage around a farmyard.

7. True or False: "Grass-fed" beef means beef from cattle raised entirely on grass.

Quiz courtesy of *Going Against GMOs* by Melissa Diane Smith.
Feel free to copy and distribute this page for education purposes.

Answers to the Quiz:

1. **False.** In order for a food manufacturer to be able to use the term "gluten-free" on its label, a food must contain less than 20 parts per million (ppm) gluten—a standard many gluten sensitivity experts think is too high. To choose food products with stricter standards against gluten, seek out products with symbols that show they are gluten-free certified by the Celiac Support Association or by the Gluten Intolerance Group (which is behind the Gluten-Free Certification Organization or GFCO). These organizations have programs that certify foods that test below 5 or 10 ppm, respectively.

2. **False.** The Food Allergen Labeling and Consumer Protection Act requires food manufacturers to identify only those allergens that are in the ingredients of the product, not allergens that might also be present in the manufacturing facility and might be picked up in the food through cross-contact. Some manufacturers voluntarily disclose the allergens that are present in their facilities. But others do not and they are not required by law to do so. If you have severe food allergies and don't see a facility allergen statement on the label, don't assume the facility is allergen free. Rather, contact a company directly to check what allergens may be in its facility.

3. **True.** The law requires that food labels identify the food source names of all these eight major allergens used to make the food. When the usual name of an ingredient (e.g., buttermilk) is a major food source name (i.e., milk), that qualifies. Otherwise, the name of the food source of a major food allergen must appear in parentheses following the name of the ingredient.

   Example: "lecithin (soy)," "flour (wheat)," and "whey (milk)"

   Or the name of the allergen food source must immediately appear after or next to the list of ingredients in a "contains" statement.

   Example: "Contains Wheat, Milk, and Soy."

4. **False.** This is one of the biggest misconceptions out there. Meat, poultry, and egg products labeled "natural" must be minimally processed and contain no artificial ingredients, but the term does not indicate how animals were raised or, in the case of plants, how they were grown. Furthermore, in a move that's exceedingly frustrating to non-GMO advocates, the FDA has declined to determine whether foods containing genetically modified ingredients may be labeled as "Natural," "All Natural" or "100% Natural." The FDA also has declined to give an official definition of "natural" to use in food labeling. However, the FDA has not objected to the use of the term if the food does not contain added color, artificial flavors, or synthetic substances. What this means to shoppers is products labeled "natural" can and often do contain GMOs, pesticides and other ingredients that people normally assume would not be in truly natural foods.

5. **True.** All those agricultural methods are excluded from organic farming. Before a food product can be labeled "USDA organic," a government-approved certifier inspects the farm where the food is grown to make sure the farmer is following those organic rules. In the case of organic meat, poultry, eggs, and dairy products, they must come from animals that are fed organic feed and are not given antibiotics or growth hormones.

6. **False.** Contrary to what most shoppers assume, in order to label chicken or eggs "free range," food producers only have to offer the chickens "access to the outside," according to the USDA. The term unfortunately doesn't mean the chickens are freely prancing around outside.

7. **False.** Grass-fed animals receive a majority of their nutrients from grass throughout their life, but they still could be fattened up on grain. To get meat from animals that are fed grass their entire lives and have numerous nutritional benefits, look for meat that is labeled both grass fed and grass finished, or 100% grass fed. To get beef from cattle raised on organic grass, look for meat that is labeled organic and 100% grass fed.

Appendix E:
Non-GMO Supplements

Some people go to great lengths to take GM foods out of their diet only to find that they are feeling unwell because they are using a supplement that is produced with GM ingredients. Be an informed shopper by studying the list of hidden GMOs in Appendix A and seeing if any of those ingredients are in vitamins you're taking. Then call or write the manufacturers and ask if those supplements contain any genetically modified ingredients such as corn, soy, sugar, and milk. You may know more about the topic than the person answering your questions, so follow up by asking educated questions about hidden GM ingredients.

You can also seek out a Non-GMO Project Verified supplement. Look for supplements from the following companies. Most if not all varieties of the vitamin, mineral, or multi-vitamin supplements made by the following manufacturers are Non-GMO Project Verified:

- **Garden of Life Kind Organics and Vitamin Code brands** (Gardenoflife.com)

- **MegaFood** (Megafood.com)

- **New Chapter** (Newchapter.com)

- **NutriGold** (Nutrigold.com)

- **TraceMinerals Research** (Traceminerals.com)

A long list of products from other manufacturers are in the process of being verified. For a current list, go to NonGMOProject.org and search in the Vitamins & Supplements category.

Appendix F:

Organic and Non-GMO Dog and Cat Foods

Pets are not only our friends but an integral part of our families, so it shouldn't be surprising that more pet owners are joining the non-GMO movement. As I described in Chapter 3, people who feed their dogs and cats non-GMO food often see their pets recovering from numerous health conditions that weren't being helped by natural remedies or veterinarian treatment.

When searching for non-GMO pet foods, understand that some pet foods that say "made with naturally GMO-free ingredients" do not contain any direct sources of GMOs, but they harbor indirect sources from conventional meat. However, dog and cat foods that are labeled USDA Organic contain 95 percent or more organic ingredients and use organic meat.

Also, bear in mind that just as cats and dogs are not adapted to eating GM foods, they also are not adapted to eating grain—and often experience dramatic improvements in many health conditions when they are given grain-free food. This is especially true of cats, which are classified as true carnivores. Dogs are mostly carnivores. In the wild, both of them eat meat from live prey, little plant material, and no grain. Though dogs may be able to utilize carbohydrates from plant foods slightly better than cats, neither cats nor dogs are metabolically adapted to high amounts of carbohydrates or grains. For the best health results with your pets, when possible, purchase organic and/or Non-GMO Project Verified pet food that is also grain free or at least gluten free.

While not a complete list, the following are some organic pet foods to look for:

- **Original Pet Food Company dog and cat food**—the first line of dog and cat food made from organic, grass-fed beef (OriginalPetFood.com)

- **Organix organic dog and cat food by Castor & Pollux Natural Petworks** (CastorPolluxPet.com)

- **Newman's Own Organics dog and cat food** (NewmansOwnOrganics.com)

- **Party Animal Organic dog and cat food** (PartyAnimalPetFood.com)

As of the date of publication of this book, there are two Non-GMO Project Verified pet foods currently on the market:

- **Mary's Organic Pet Food**

- **The Furry Foodie raw frozen organic complete meals for dogs and cats** (TheFurryFoodie.com)

Other companies are enrolled in the Non-GMO Project program and in the process of being verified. For the latest information, visit NonGMOProject.org or NonGMOShoppingGuide.com. Look for non-GMO pet products in natural food stores or shop online at Organic-Pet-Food.com, ShopOrganic.com, and Amazon.com.

Appendix G:
GMO Boycotting and Banning vs. Labeling

Getting honest, complete information about what's in the food we're considering buying seems like such a basic right, it isn't surprising that more than 90 percent of Americans support the labeling of GMOs in food. It also isn't surprising why so many people have fought, and continue to fight, for labeling. I truly wish genetically modified foods had not been allowed on the market or at least had been labeled so people had a clear choice about whether to eat them from the beginning. That unfortunately didn't happen. Now, after much consideration, I feel the situation with GM foods in the United States and Canada has gone simply too far and I believe that our efforts should be focused on boycotting and banning GMOs.

It boils down to this: *In our country, large agrichemical corporations have so much power that the conditions are stacked against us getting honest, truthful labeling, checking, and policing of GM foods.* The history of what has happened with other types of labeling shows us this is true, as I'll soon explain. In addition, while many people are working hard for labeling on a state-by-state basis, GMOs continue to spread through wind drift and contaminate conventional and organic crops.

WHY I CHANGED MY OPINION

Even when I knew only some of the hazards of GM foods, I was *against GMOs* being in our food supply at all and I wanted to avoid GMOs in what I ate and have my clients and the public also be able to easily avoid GMOs to protect their health. Therefore, *I was automatically "for labeling" without thinking about it.*

However, as a nutritionist with many clients with food allergies and gluten intolerance, I have observed what has happened with first "food allergen-free" labeling and then "gluten-free" labeling. What I have seen is that each time labeling is enacted, the standards that are developed favor industry over people's health, allowing a little bit of the allergens in allergen-free foods, no checking or enforcing of the guidelines, and food companies policing themselves, which some companies, perhaps many companies, don't do at all. The label regulations are weak, which puts consumers at risk. Consider the following two examples.

EXAMPLES FROM OTHER TYPES OF LABELING

The food allergen labeling law was passed in 2004. In 2008, a *Chicago Tribune* special investigation found that lack of testing and policing of food allergens leads to allergic people and kids often having reactions that send them to the hospital from "allergen-free" foods that aren't really free of those allergens. Often little disciplinary action is taken against the companies whose products are mislabeled.

With gluten free, the situation was slightly different: People fought for close to a decade for gluten-free labeling of foods. Since there was no definitive ruling at the federal level about what constituted "gluten free," people who were adamant about avoiding gluten didn't wait for federal action. Instead, they ended up being proactive, calling companies to directly ask them if their products contained gluten. If the products did contain gluten, customers asked the manufacturers to change to gluten-free ingredients.

The grassroots activism by gluten-sensitive people convinced food manufacturers that there was such a demand for gluten-free foods that the companies better start offering what people want or they would lose many customers. That consumer activism changed the marketplace and gluten free became big business—such big business that the FDA finally got into the act and came up with its ruling on what "gluten free" means in 2013. To the great dismay of practitioners like myself who are aware of the many health problems that occur when gluten-sensitive people eat even small amounts of gluten, the FDA's decision on "gluten free" ended up being weak: It favors industry over people's health and it does not really mean free of gluten.

Supposedly, the idea is that a state GMO labeling initiative would put the power in the hands of the public more. However, when enough state bills are passed, consumers, companies, and the government will all have to come to the table to negotiate for federal labeling. The first thing that will happen when those talks start to occur is state actions will be pre-empted to get labeling at the federal level. According to one legislative spokesperson I heard, "compromises will need to be made."

From my viewpoint, there is no evidence that the outcomes from GMO labeling efforts will end up better than what happened with efforts for other types of labeling in recent years. What is different and particularly frightening about GMOs is that GMOs, unlike food allergens or gluten, are life forms that spread and contaminate other similar crops. *For that reason, the issue of taking the right action against GMOs is so critical for protecting our environment and the future of our food, we simply can't afford to spend our time and energy on efforts that are ineffective at achieving what we want.*

WHY FOCUS ON BOYCOTTS AND BANS?

There are two efforts that will give us the most bang for the buck in stopping GMOs in our food supply. The first is to be real consumer activists, starting out by following my Eat GMO-Free Challenge in Chapter 7, and then getting even more proactive by calling companies, writing letters, and telling companies you won't buy any more of their products until they take the GMOs out. Trust me: if enough consumers say no, the companies will respond to the demand or go out of business. We shouldn't be "on hold" waiting for labeling. We have all the information we need right now to stop buying and eating GMOs. That's exactly why I created the Eat GMO-Free Challenge and wrote this book to get consumers to individually and collectively use their consumer power.

The second way to be effective, particularly against the disturbing issue of GMOs spreading and contaminating more and more food, is to focus our efforts on bans or at the very least moratoriums. (If you're wondering the difference, a ban prohibits the planting of GM crops, whereas a moratorium puts a temporary prohibition on the planting of GM crops, usually for a specific period of years.)

The first step in achieving this is to believe we can. We already know it's possible: Other countries, such as Mexico and Peru, have passed bans and moratoriums, and as I explained in Chapter 14, several counties in the western United States have successfully passed countywide bans in recent years on the planting of GM crops. To accomplish that more frequently and eventually put a halt to the growing of GM crops in our country, we have to believe in the tremendous power we have as consumers and citizens.

If you have been firmly "for GMO labeling," consider what I have written here. I say: Focus on avoiding GMOs in the shopping you do now, and find others to work with to accomplish more bans against GMOs. GM foods are such a serious issue, with so many potentially harmful consequences to our food, health, and planet, we literally have no time to waste.

Resources

I've listed films, books, and websites in what I consider priority order. If you don't know where to begin learning additional information, consider starting at the top of each category's list.

Film Documentaries on GM Foods

Genetic Roulette: The Gamble of Our Lives (85 minutes) – www.geneticroulettemovie.com

A groundbreaking, award-winning documentary about the health dangers of GMOs by Jeffrey M. Smith. The film explains how GM foods are a gamble unprecedented in all of history and ties the increase in a variety of common diseases and disorders to our eating untested GM foods.

The Future of Food (88 minutes) – www.thefutureoffood.com

An in-depth investigation into the disturbing truth behind unlabeled, patented, genetically engineered foods that have quietly filled grocery store shelves. This movie was released in 2004, but the information it covers holds up well and thoroughly explains the serious problems associated with GM foods.

Hidden Dangers in Kids' Meals (28 minutes) – available from www.seedsofdeception.com

This older but still very informative film explains, in a short period of time, why GM foods are dangerous and should be removed from our and our kids' meals—and why growing children may be the most vulnerable to their effects.

Deconstructing Supper (48 minutes) – available from www.bullfrogfilms.com

A film that follows the journey of an acclaimed chef who learns about GMOs, the huge change in modern food production, its effects on our lives, and the importance of growing food organically. I consider this a gentle introduction to the topic of genetically engineered foods.

Film Documentaries on Recent Changes to Our Food System

King Corn (88 minutes) – www.kingcorn.net

A feature documentary about two friends, one acre of corn, and the subsidized crop that drives our fast-food nation. Best friends from college move to the heartland to plant and grow this heavily subsidized crop. When they try to follow their pile of corn into the food system, what they find raises troubling questions about how we eat and how we farm.

Fed Up (92 minutes) – www.fedupmovie.com

A 2014 documentary that explains that everything we've been told about food and exercise the past 30 years is wrong. It presents evidence showing that the large quantities of sugar in processed foods are an overlooked root of the problem and points to the moneyed lobbying power of "Big Sugar" in blocking attempts to enact effective policies to address the issue.

Food, Inc. (94 minutes) – More info at www.takepart.com

A film that lifts the veil on our nation's food industry, exposing the mechanized underbelly that has been hidden from the American consumer with the consent of our government's regulatory agencies, the USDA and FDA, and how our nation's food supply is now controlled by a handful of corporations that put profit ahead of consumer health, the livelihood of the American farmer, the safety of workers, and our own environment.

Unacceptable Levels (76 minutes) – www.unacceptablelevels.com

From the products we use, to the food we eat, to the air we breathe, this film documents how prevalent toxic chemicals have become in our lives and why we must do something about it.

Reports & Books for More Information on GMOs

GMO Myths and Truths—at www.Earthopensource.org

This report, available as a free online download by the sustainability and science policy platform Earth Open Source, is an evidence-based examination of the claims made for the safety and efficacy of GM crops.

Your Right to Know: Genetic Engineering and the Secret Changes in Your Food by Andrew Kimbrell

A comprehensive guide and informative coffee table book about GM foods and how they are impacting our lives written by the executive director of the Center for Food Safety.

Seeds of Deception: Exposing Industry and Government Lies about the Safety of the Genetically Engineered Foods You're Eating by Jeffrey M. Smith

An investigative book with stories that reveal how industry manipulation and political collusion allowed GM foods on the market without labeling.

Genetic Roulette: The Documented Health Risks of Genetically Engineered Foods by Jeffrey M. Smith

An easy-to-browse guide that outlines 65 health risks based on studies on GM foods as well as suppressed science and cover-ups.

The Unhealthy Truth by Robyn O'Brien

A first-person story from a mother who researched recent changes in our food system after her child had a severe allergic reaction. The book reveals the alarming relationship between the manipulation of our food with more additives and GM ingredients and recent increases in allergies, ADHD, cancer, and asthma among our children.

Birke on the Farm: The Story of a Boy's Search for Real Food by Birke Baehr

An easy-to-read picture book that tells the story of a boy's journey of discovery about food and farming. The book is designed to help small children learn about the food system.

My Previous Nutrition Books

Going Against the Grain: How Reducing and Avoiding Grains Can Revitalize Your Health by Melissa Diane Smith
More than a dozen years in print, this groundbreaking book challenges conventional dietary wisdom—that grains should be the centerpiece of our diet—and presents scientific information in easy-to-understand terms on the surprising nutritional problems of grains—and the grain connection to conditions such as obesity, diabetes, Syndrome X, auto-immune disorders, celiac disease, gluten sensitivity, grain allergies, and digestive problems.

Gluten Free Throughout the Year by Melissa Diane Smith
With more than 100 tips, 30 recipes, and names of the healthiest gluten-free food brands and products, this is an easy-to-read, tip-based practical guide for living a healthy gluten-free lifestyle.

Syndrome X: The Complete Nutritional Program to Prevent and Reverse Insulin Resistance by Jack Challem, Burton Berkson, and Melissa Diane Smith
A national bestselling book that explains, in simple terms, how the prediabetic condition Syndrome X (also known as metabolic syndrome) develops. The condition is the combination of insulin resistance with extra weight around the middle, unhealthy cholesterol ratios, high tri-glycerides, and/or high blood pressure that ages people prematurely and sets the stage for heart disease, type 2 diabetes and other common degenerative diseases.

Websites for More Information on My Work

MelissaDianeSmith.com
My website with information on my background, books, speaking services, and long-distance nutrition consultations and coaching programs that I conduct over the phone.

AgainstTheGrainNutrition.com

My website to spread the word about the healing power of Against the Grain Nutrition, which of course includes avoiding GMOs. You can use the search engine on the blog to look for up-to-date, in-depth articles on genetically modified foods, as well as gluten sensitivity, celiac disease, insulin resistance, overweight, type 2 diabetes, and the benefits of gluten-free and grain-free diets.

EatGMOFreeChallenge.com

My series of 31 tips to help you learn how to avoid GMOs, which are also in Chapter 7 of this book. On this website page, you can click to view just one tip at a time.

Websites for More Information on Non-GMO Shopping

Non-GMO Project – NonGMOProject.org

A non-profit organization that offers North America's only third party verification and labeling for non-GMO food and products. Search through the website to find the most up-to-date list of Non-GMO Project Verified products.

Non-GMO Shopping Guide – NonGMOShoppingGuide.com

A consumer-oriented site produced by the Institute for Responsible Technology where you can view or download a free Non-GMO Shopping Guide or get the mobile application for the iPhone.

Center for Food Safety – CenterforFoodSafety.org

Search for the True Food Shopper's Guide and download the guide or get the mobile application for iPhone and Android.

Shop Organic & Shop GMO Free – ShopOrganic.com

A women-owned small mail-order business at which you can purchase a wide variety of organic and GMO-free products.

High Mowing Organic Seeds – HighMowingSeeds.com

The first Non-GMO Project Verified seed company; an organic seed company closely involved with the Open Source Seed Initiative.

Websites for More Information on Organic Shopping

Organic Consumers Association – OrganicConsumers.org.

Search for tips for organic on a budget.

Environmental Working Group – Ewg.org/foodnews.

Enter your email address to download the Shopper's Guide to Pesticides in Produce or get the App for your smart phone.

Websites for General Information about GM Foods

Institute for Responsible Technology – ResponsibleTechnology.org

A world leader in educating policy makers and the public about GM foods and crops and their risks and impact on health, the environment, the economy, and agriculture.

Center for Food Safety – CenterforFoodSafety.org

A national non-profit organization that works to protect human health and the environment by curbing the proliferation of harmful food production technologies, by promoting organic and other forms of sustainable agriculture, and by engaging in legal, scientific and grassroots initiatives to guide national and international policymaking on critical food safety issues.

Organic Consumers Association – OrganicConsumers.org

A grassroots non-profit organization that focuses on crucial issues of food safety, industrial agriculture, genetic engineering, corporate accountability, and environmental sustainability.

Food Democracy Now – Fooddemocracy.org

A grassroots movement of more than 650,000 farmers and citizens dedicated to reforming policies related to food and agriculture and to building a sustainable food system that protects our natural environment, sustains farmers, and nourishes families. You can learn more about the Monsanto Stock Plunge campaign at this site.

Food Integrity Now – Foodintegritynow.org

A site with more than 100 podcasts featuring outstanding guests influencing positive change and integrity in the global food supply. The site's goal is to provide accurate and timely information on food and health-related issues, including offering a wealth of information on GMOs.

Friends of the Earth – Foe.org

A network of grassroots groups in 74 countries that defend the environment and champion a more healthy and just world.

GMO Free USA – GMOFreeUSA.com

A national group that leads campaigns and boycotts involving hundreds of thousands of non-GMO activists to collectively speak to and influence large U.S. food manufacturers to remove GMOs from the products they sell.

GMO Inside – GMOInside.org

A coalition of individuals and organizations dedicated to helping Americans know which foods have GMOs inside, and the non-GMO verified and organic certified alternatives to GM foods.

The Organic and Non-GMO Report – Non-GMOReport.com

A news magazine that provides up-to-date, easy-to-understand information about organic and non-GMO products, GMO food issues, how to prevent GMO contamination, and more.

Websites for Parent-Oriented Information

Spoonfed – Spoonfed.com

An engaging website and blog written by journalist and mother Christina Le Beau about raising kids to think about the food they eat. It has a helpful list of resources for parents getting started in the process of understanding real food and raising food-literate kids.

Allergy Kids – AllergyKids.com

Founded by *The Unhealthy Truth* author Robyn O'Brien, Allergy Kids' goal is to protect children from the additives now found in our food supply—additives not used in children's foods in other developed countries. This is another good source of practical, supportive information for parents starting the transition to more GMO-free foods.

Moms Across America – MomsAcrossAmerica.com

A national coalition of moms whose intention is to raise awareness, share information about how moms have seen their kids' health improve going GMO free and organic, and support moms with solutions to eat GMO free.

Websites for Youth-Oriented Information

Birke on the Farm – BirkeOnTheFarm.com

The official website of youth non-GMO/organic advocate and speaker Birke Baehr, author of *Birke on the Farm: The Story of a Boy's Search for Real Food.* You can purchase his book and view speeches and interviews with Birke on this site.

Kids Right to Know – KidsRightToKnow.com

A blog by teen activist Rachel Parent's Right to Know group that is designed to educate and inform youth about GM food, nutrition, health, and environmental and social issues affecting us all today.

References

Introduction

[1] Regal, Phillip J. Deaths and Cripplings from Genetically Engineered L-trytophan. *Seeds of Deception*, http://www.seedsofdeception.com/utility/showArticle/?objectID=277.

[2] Franck C, SM Grandi, and MJ Eisenberg. Agricultural Subsidies and the American Obesity Epidemic. *American Journal of Preventive Medicine*, 2013 Sep;45(3):327-33. doi: 10.1016/j.amepre.2013.04.010.

[3] Mercola, Joseph. U.S. Farm Subsidy Policies Contribute to Worsening Obesity Trends. *Mercola* (blog), July 27, 2013. http://articles.mercola.com/sites/articles/archive/2013/07/27/us-farm-subsidies.aspx.

Chapter 1

[4] Westgate, Megan. Non-GMO Project Moves to Expand Verification Capabilities. *Non-GMO Project* (blog), September 17, 2013. http://www.nongmoproject.org/2013/09/17/non-gmo-project-moves-to-expand-verification-capabilities/.

[5] Kinsman, Caroline, Non-GMO Project Communications Director. Email reply to the author, October 29, 2013.

[6] Beecher, Cookson. Whole Foods to Require Labeling of GMO Foods. *Food Safety News,* March 15, 2013. http://www.foodsafetynews.com/2013/03/whole-foods-to-require-labeling-of-gmo-foods/#.Um_xHCQh07A.

[7] Non-GMO Foods Are In the Spotlight, According to Latest Packaged Facts Report. *PR Web*, September 24, 2013. http://www.prweb.com/releases/2013/9/prweb11129235.htm.

[8] Marshall, Lisa. Organic Continues Double-Digit Gains. *NFM Market Overview,* May 31, 2013. http://newhope360.com/nfm-market-overview/organic-continues-double-digit-gains.

[9] Roseboro, Ken. Does Non-GMO Compete with Organic? *Delicious Living,* July 9, 2013. http://m.deliciousliving.com/nutrition/does-non-gmo-compete-organic.

[10] Weise, Elizabeth. Kashi's Cereal's 'Natural' Claims Stir Anger. *USA Today,* April 29, 2012. http://www.usatoday.com/money/industries/food/story/2012-04-29/kashi-natural-claims/54616576/1.

[11] Angry Consumers Deluge Kashi with Concerns over GMO Subterfuge. The Cornucopia Institute. *Cornucopia News,* April 26, 2012. http://www.cornucopia.org/2012/04/angry-consumers-deluge-kashi-with-concerns-over-gmo-subterfuge/.

[12] Kashi. Our Non-GMO Project Verified Commitment. http://www.kashi.com/ourcommitment.

[13] Rhodan, Maya. General Mills to Sell GMO-Free Cheerios. *TIME,* January 3, 2014. http://business.time.com/2014/01/03/general-mills-to-sell-gmo-free-cheerios/.

[14] Horovitz, Bruce. Cheerios Drops Genetically Modified Ingredients. *USA Today,* January 2, 2014. http://www.usatoday.com/story/money/business/2014/01/02/cheerios-gmos-cereals/4295739/.

[15] Watson, Elaine. Post Unveils Non-GMO Verified Grape Nuts as Gen Mills Says Goodbye to GMOs in Original Cheerios. *Food Navigator-USA,* January 17, 2014. http://www.foodnavigator-usa.com/Manufacturers/Post-unveils-non-GMO-verified-Grape-Nuts-as-Gen-Mills-says-goodbye-to-GMOs-in-Original-Cheerios.

[16] GMO Inside Congratulates Post on Non-GMO Grape Nuts. *GMO Inside* (blog), January 16, 2014. http://gmoinside.org/gmo-inside-congratulates-post-non-gmo-grape-nuts/.

[17] Robb, Walter, and A.C. Gallo. GMO Labeling Coming to Whole Foods Market. *Whole Foods Market* (blog), March 8, 2013. http://www.wholefoodsmarket.com/blog/gmo-labeling-coming-whole-foods-market.

[18] Strom, Stephanie. Food Companies Seeking Ingredients That Aren't Gene-Altered. *The New York Times,* May 27, 2013. http://www.nytimes.com/2013/05/27/business/food-companies-seeking-ingredients-that-arent-gene-altered.html?pagewanted=all.

[19] Roseboro, Ken. Chipotle Commits to Going Non-GMO. *Organic Connection.* http://organicconnectmag.com/chipotle-commits-going-non-gmo/#.UsjPp_Yh07A.

[20] O'Brien, Robyn. Wall Street's Leading Indicator: A Non GMO Burrito. *RobynOBrien* (blog), January 2, 2014. http://www.robynobrien.com/_blog/ Inspiring_Ideas/post/wall-streets-leading-indicator-a-non-gmo-burrito/.

[21] Frias, Arnold. Hedge Funds Are Dumping Monsanto Company (MON). *Insider Monkey,* August 21, 2013. http://www.insidermonkey.com/blog/ hedge-funds-are-dumping-monsanto-company-mon-224412/

[22] Food Democracy Now. Campaigns: Take the Monsanto Stock Plunge page. http://action.fooddemocracynow.org/sign/take_the_Monsanto_stock_plunge/.

[23] Adams, Mike. Monsanto, biotech stocks plummet the day after activists launch Operation Monsanto Stock Plunge. *Natural News,* April 11, 2014. http://www.naturalnews.com/044672_biotech_stocks_market_plunge_ monsanto.html.

[24] Schweigert, Mary Beth. How GMOs Impact the GF Diet: Frequent Use of Corn and Soy Raises Questions. *Gluten-Free Living,* February 2014, pgs. 28-31.

[25] Kopicki, Allison. Strong Support for Labeling Modified Foods. *The New York Times,* July 27, 2013. http://www.nytimes.com/2013/07/28/science/ strong-support-for-labeling-modified-foods.html?_r=0.

[26] The NPD Group. Over Half of U.S. Consumers Concerned about Genetically-Modified Foods, But the Definition of GMOs is Unclear among Consumers, Reports NPD. *PR Web,* December 19, 2013. http://www.prweb. com/releases/2013/12/prweb11436077.htm.

Chapter 2

[27] Druker, Steven M. How the U.S. Food and Drug Administration Approved Genetically Engineered Foods Despite the Deaths One Had Caused and the Warnings of Its Own Scientists about Their Unique Risks. Alliance for Bio-Integrity. http://www.biointegrity.org/ext-summary.htm.

[28] Mellman, Mark. Majority want more labels on food. *The Mellman Group,* April 17, 2012. http://www.mellmangroup.com/index.php?option=com_conte nt&view=article&id=531:majority-want-more-labels-on-food&catid=40:com mentary&Itemid=96.

[29] Just Label It! website. Just Label It! Right to Know web page. http:// justlabelit.org/right-to-know/.

[30] Murphy, Dave. 20 Years of GMO Policy That Keeps Americans in the Dark About Their Food. *The Huffington Post,* May 30, 2012. http://www. huffingtonpost.com/dave-murphy/dan-quayle-and-michael-ta_b_1551732. html.

[31] From Dan Quayle to Obama: The Politics of GMOs: Interview with Dave Murphy, by Stacy Malkan. GMOs: What You Need to Know Online Conference, January 29, 2014.

[32] Antoniou, Michael, Claire Robinson, and John Fagan. GMO Myths and Truths: An Evidence-Based Examination of the Claims Made for the Safety and Efficacy of Genetically Modified Crops, version 1.3. Earth Open Source, June 2012. http://earthopensource.org/index.php/reports/gmo-myths-and-truths.

[33] Bartolotto, Carole, M.A., R.D. Is the Movement to Label GMOs Anti-Science? *Healthy Eating Rocks!* June 14, 2013. http://healthyeatingrocks. com/2013/06/14/is-the-movement-to-label-gmos-anti-science/.

[34] The Science of GMOs and Unintended Consequences: Interview with Michael Hansen, Ph.D., by Stacy Malkan. GMOs: What You Need to Know Online Conference, January 27, 2014.

[35] Smith, Jeffrey M. *Genetic Roulette: The Documented Health Risks of Genetically Engineered Foods.* Fairfield, Iowa: Yes! Books. 2007, pgs. 1-2.

[36] Hansen, Michael. Phone interview with the author, April 4, 2014.

[37] Bello, Walden, and Foreign Policy in Focus. Twenty-Six Countries Ban GMOs—Why Won't the U.S.? *The Nation,* October 29, 2013. http://www. thenation.com/blog/176863/twenty-six-countries-ban-gmos-why-wont-us.

[38] Kimbrell, Andrew. *Your Right to Know: Genetic Engineering and the Secret Changes in Your Food.* San Rafael, CA: Earth Aware, 2007, pg. 48.

[39] Benbrook, Charles. Impacts of Genetically Engineered Crops on Pesticide Use—The First Sixteen Years. *Environmental Sciences Europe* 2012, 24:24 doi:10.1186/2190-4715-24-24. http://www.enveurope.com/content/24/1/24/ abstract.

[40] Freese, Bill. Going Backwards: Dow's 2,4-D-Resistant Crops and a More Toxic Future. *Food Safety Review,* Winter 2012, pgs. 1-4.

[41] Pollack, Andrew. Dow Corn, Resistant to a Weed Killer, Runs into Opposition. *The New York Times,* April 25, 2012, http://www.nytimes.com/2012/04/26/business/energy-environment/dow-weed-killer-runs-into-opposition.html?pagewanted=all.

[42] Benbrook, Charles. *Environmental Sciences Europe.* Op cit.

[43] Tabashnik BE, T Brevault, and Y Carriere. Insect Resistance in Bt Crops: Lessons from the First Billion Acres. *Nature Biotechnology* 2013 Jun;31(6):510-21. doi: 10.1038/nbt.2597.

[44] Upton, John. Five Pest Species Now Immune to GMO Corn and Cotton. *Grist,* June 13, 2013. http://grist.org/news/five-pest-species-now-immune-to-gmo-corn-and-cotton/.

[45] Antoniou, Michael, et al. GMO Myths and Truths. Op cit.

[46] Pesticide Action Network North America. Pesticides 101: A Primer. http://www.panna.org/issues/pesticides-101-primer#2.

[47] Gurian-Sherman, Doug. Failure to Yield: Evaluating the Performance of Genetically Engineered Crops. Union of Concerned Scientists, April 14, 2009. http://www.ucsusa.org/food_and_agriculture/science_and_impacts/science/failure-to-yield.html.

[48] Elmore RW, FW Roeth, LA Nelson, et al. Glyphosate-Resistant Soyabean Cultivar Yields Compared with Sister Lines. *Agronomy Journal,* 93: 408-412, 2001.

[49] Heinemann JA, M Massaro, DS Coray, et al. Sustainability and Innovation in Staple Crop Production in the U.S. Midwest. *International Journal of Agricultural Sustainability,* 2013, doi: 10.1080/14735903.2013.806408.

[50] University of Canterbury Researchers: GM is a Failing Technology. *SustainablePulse,* June 20, 2013. http://sustainablepulse.com/2013/06/20/university-of-canterbury-researchers-gm-is-a-failing-biotechnology/#.U_Usi0hNc7A.

[51] Kimbrell. Andrew. Phone interview with the author, May 29, 2012.

[52] *The Future of Food* [documentary]. Directed by Deborah Koons Garcia. Lily Films, 2004.

[53] Saved Seed and Farmer Lawsuits. Monsanto website. http://www.monsanto.com/newsviews/pages/saved-seed-farmer-lawsuits.aspx.

[54] Farmers vs. Monsanto page. *Food Democracy Now!* http://www.fooddemocracynow.org/farmers-vs-monsanto.

[55] Who Owns Nature? Corporate Power and the Final Frontier in the Commodification of Life. ETC *Group Communique,* November 2008, Issue #100. http://www.etcgroup.org/content/who-owns-nature.

[56] The World's Top 10 Seed Companies: Who Owns Nature? *GM Watch.* http://www.gmwatch.org/gm-firms/10558-the-worlds-top-ten-seed-companies-who-owns-nature.

[57] Who Do You Trust to Control Our Food Choices?: Interview with Zack Kaldveer, Ph.D., by Stacy Malkan. GMOs: What You Need to Know Online Conference, January 30, 2014.

[58] Strassmann, Paul. *Frontline.* The Pernicious Characteristics of Monocultures. http://www.pbs.org/wgbh/pages/frontline/shows/hackers/blame/threat.html.

[59] Organic Consumers Association Email. Urgent Deadline: Tell the USDA: No GMO Apple. December 12, 2013.

[60] Food Democracy Now! Email. GMO Kiss of Death Apple. December 13, 2013.

[61] Center for Food Safety Email. Last Chance to Comment Against GE Apples. January 28, 2014.

[62] Target, Giant Eagle, H-E-B, Meijer Say No to Genetically Engineered Salmon. *Center for Food Safety* (press release), May 29, 2013. http://www.centerforfoodsafety.org/press-releases/2249/target-giant-eagle-h-e-b-meijer-say-no-to-genetically-engineered-salmon.

[63] Environmental Groups Take Federal Government to Court for Permitting Manufacture of Genetically Modified Salmon in Canada. *Ecojustice* (press release), January 20, 2013. http://www.ecojustice.ca/media-centre/press-releases/environmental-groups-take-federal-government-to-court-for-permitting-manufacture-of-genetically-modified-salmon-in-canada.

[64] Vennare, Martin. Can Genetically Modified Mosquitoes Prevent Disease in the U.S.? *BBC News,* January 4, 2013.

[65] Sierra Club. Genetic Engineering: Genetically Engineered Trees. http://vault.sierraclub.org/biotech/trees.aspx.

[66] *A Silent Forest: The Growing Threat, Genetically Engineered Trees* [documentary]. Directed by Ed Schehl. Three Americas, Inc., 2009.

[67] Center for Food Safety. *Genetically Engineered Trees: The New Frontier of Biotechnology* report, November 2013. http://www.centerforfoodsafety.org/reports/2637/genetically-engineered-trees-the-new-frontier-of-biotechnology.

[68] Leschin-Hoar, Clare. Fed Help GMO Salmon Swim Upstream. *Grist,* September 29, 2011. http://grist.org/food/2011-09-29-feds-help-gmo-salmon-swim-upstream/,

[69] Fed Grant $500K to Genetically Engineered Livestock Research. *Sustainable Food News,* December 26, 2012. http://www.sustainablefoodnews.com/story.php?news_id=18142.

[70] *The Future of Food* [documentary]. Op. cit.

[71] U.S. Food and Drug Administration. Meet Michael R. Taylor, J.D., Deputy Commissioner for Foods and Veterinary Medicine. http://www.fda.gov/aboutfda/centersoffices/officeoffoods/ucm196721.htm.

Chapter 3

[72] *Scientists Under Attack: Genetic Engineering in the Magnetic Field of Money* [documentary]. Directed by Bertram Verhaag. DENKmal-Films Ltd., 2009.

[73] *Genetic Roulette: The Gamble of Our Lives* [documentary]. Directed by Jeffrey Smith. Fairfield, IA: The Institute for Responsible Technology, 2012.

[74] The American Academy of Environmental Medicine Calls for Immediate Moratorium on Genetically Modified Foods. *American Academy of Environmental Medicine* (press release), May 19, 2009. http://www.aaemonline.org/gmopressrelease.html.

[75] Genetically Modified Foods. *American Academy of Environmental Medicine.* http://www.aaemonline.org/gmopost.html.

[76] Séralini GE, et al. Long term toxicity of a Roundup herbicide and a Roundup-tolerant genetically modified maize. *Food and Chemical Toxicity.* (2012), http://dx.doi.org/10.1016/j.fct.2012.08.005.

[77] ISIS, Institute of Science in Society. Scientists Pledge to Boycott Elsevier. *The Ecologist,* December 5, 2013. http://www.theecologist.org/blogs_and_comments/commentators/2187010/scientists_pledge_to_boycott_elsevier.html.

[78] Séralini GE, Clair E, Mesnage R, et al. Republished study: long-term toxicity of a Roundup herbicide and a Roundup-tolerant genetically modified maize. *Environmental Sciences Europe* 2014, 26:14 doi:10.1186/s12302-014-0014-5.

[79] *Genetic Roulette* [documentary film], 2012, op cit.

[80] Carman JA, HR Vlieger, LJ Ver Steeg, et al. A Long-Term Toxicology Study on Pigs Fed a Combined Genetically Modified (GM) Soy and GM Maize Diet. *Journal of Organic Systems,* 2013, 8(1):38-54.

[81] Ewen, Stanley W. B., and A Pusztai . Effects of Diets Containing Genetically Modified Potatoes Expressing Galanthus nivalis Lectin on Rat Small Intestine. *Lancet,* 1999 Oct 16; 354 (9187):1353-4.

[82] Smith, Jeffrey. Compelling Stories about Our Non-GMO National Movement. *Institute for Responsible Technology* (blog), November 26, 2013, http://www.responsibletechnology.org/posts/compelling-stories-about-our-national-non-gmo-movement/.

[83] Vrain, Thierry. Former Pro-GMO Scientist Speaks Out On The Real Dangers of Genetically Engineered Food. The Food Revolution Network (blog), May 11, 2013. http://foodrevolution.org/blog/former-pro-gmo-scientist/.

[84] From Pro GMO to Anti GMO: Interview with Thierry Vrain, Ph.D., by Stacy Malkan. GMOs: What You Need to Know Online Conference, January 27, 2014.

[85] Protect Your Children from Genetically Modified Foods informational brochure. Institute for Responsible Technology.

[86] Aris A, and S Leblanc. Maternal and Fetal Exposure to Pesticides Associated to Genetically Modified Foods in Eastern Townships of Quebec, Canada. *Reproductive Toxicology.* 2011 May;31(4):528-33. Epub 2011 Feb 18.

[87] Trends in Children's Health and the Path to Healing: Interview with Michello Perro, M.D., by Stacy Malkan. GMOs: What You Need to Know Online Conference, January 29, 2014.

[88] Sirinathsinghji E, and MW Ho. Why Glyphosate Should Be Banned—A Review of Its Hazard to Health and the Environment. Permaculture Research Institute. *Permaculturenews,* November 1, 2012. http://permaculturenews. org/2012/11/01/why-glyphosate-should-be-banned-a-review-of-its-hazards-to-health-and-the-environment/.

[89] Paganelli, A., V Gnazzo, H Acosta, et al. Glyphosate-based Herbicides Produce Teratogenic Effects on Vertebrates by Impairing Retinoic Acid Signalling. *Chemical Research in Toxicology,* 2010 Oct 18;23(10):1586-95. doi: 10.1021/tx1001749. Epub 2010 Aug 9.

[90] Gasnier C, C Dumont, N Benachour, et al. Glyphosate-based Herbicides are Toxic and Endocrine Disruptors in Human Cell Lines. *Toxicology.* 2009 Aug 21;262(3):184-91. doi: 10.1016/j.tox.2009.06.006. Epub 2009 Jun 17.

[91] Huber, Don. Ag Chemical and Crop Nutrient Interactions—Current Updates. Proceedings Fluid Fertilizer Forum, Scottsdale, AZ February 14-16, 2010. Vol. 27. Fluid Fertilizer Foundation, Manhattan, KS. Shared on Greenpasture.org on November 12, 2012. http://www.greenpasture.org/fermented-cod-liver-oil-butter-oil-vitamin-d-vitamin-a/important-paper-on-glyphosate---and-discussion-on-the-new-pathogen-effecting-plant-animal-and-human-fertility/?back=javascript:history.back%28%29;.

[92] Mercola, Joseph. Toxicology Expert Speaks Out About Roundup and GMOs. *Mercola,* October 6, 2013. http://articles.mercola.com/sites/articles/archive/2013/10/06/dr-huber-gmo-foods.aspx.

[93] Smith, Jeffrey. Monsanto's Roundup Triggers Over 40 Plant Diseases and Endangers Human and Animal Health. *Institute for Responsibility* (blog), January 14, 2011. http://www.responsibletechnology.org/posts/monsanto%E2%80%99s-roundup-triggers-over-40-plant-diseases/.

[94] Ibid.

[95] GMOs, Glyphosate & Tomorrow: An Interview with Don Huber, Ph.D. *ACRES USA,* May 2011, Vol. 41, No. 5. Reprinted by Organicconsumers. org, May 1, 2011. http://www.organicconsumers.org/artman2/uploads/1/May2011_Huber.pdf.

[96] Sanz Y, G De Pama, and M Laparra. Unraveling the Ties Between Celiac Disease and Intestinal Microbiota. *International Reviews of Immunology,* August 2011;30(4):207-18. doi: 10.3109/08830185.2011.599084.

[97] Tilg, Herbert, and Arthur Kaiser. Gut Microbiome, Obesity, and Metabolic Dysfunction. *Journal of Clinical Investigation,* 2011;121(6):2126-2132. doi:10.1172/JCI58109.

[98] Vazquez-Padron RI, L Moreno-Fierros, L Neri-Bazan, et al. Intragastric and Intraperitoneal Administration of Cry1Ac protoxin from *Bacillus thuringiensis* Induces Systemic and Mucosal Antibody Responses in Mice. *Life Sciences,* 1999; 64, no. 21: 1897-1912.

[99] Vazquez-Padron RI, L Moreno-Fierros, L Neri-Bazan, et al. Characterization of the Mucosal and Systemic Immune Response Induced by Cry1Ac protein from *Bacillus thuringiensis* HD 73 in Mice. *Brazilian Journal of Medical and Biological Research,* 2000; 33: 147-155.

[100] Nordlee JA, SL Taylor, JA Townsend, et al. Identification of a Brazil-nut Allergen in Transgenic Soybeans. *New England Journal of Medicine,* 1996:334: 688-92.

[101] Nestle M. Allergies to Transgenic Foods: Questions of Policy. *New England Journal of Medicine,* 1996; 334: 726-28.

[102] After the Introduction of Genetically Modified Soy, Soy Allergies Skyrocket in the UK. York Nutritional Laboratory. Press Release, March 12, 1999.

[103] Soy Allergy/Adverse Effect Rates Skyrocket—Monsanto's Roundup-Ready Soy Blamed. Soyinfo.com, March 12, 1999. http://www.soyinfo.com/allergy2.shtml.

[104] Padgette, Stephen R, et al. The Composition of Glyphosate-Tolerant Soybean Seeds is Equivalent to That of Conventional Soybeans, *Journal of Nutrition,* April 1996; 126, no. 4. In Jeffrey M. Smith. *Seeds of Deception* (Yes! Books, 2003), pg. 161.

[105] Genetically Engineering Foods May Cause Rising Food Allergies (Part One), *Spilling the Beans* by the Institute for Responsible Technology, May 2007, http://www.seedsofdeception.com/utility/showArticle/?objectID=1007.

[106] From Starlink to Salmon: The Rise of the People's Movement for Healthier Food: Interview with Lisa Archer, by Stacy Malkan. GMOs: What You Need to Know Online Conference, January 28, 2014.

[107] Food Allergy Facts and Statistics for the U.S. Food Allergy Research & Education. http://www.foodallergy.org/facts-and-stats.

[108] Trends in Children's Health and the Path to Healing: Interview with Michelle Perro, M.D., by Stacy Malkan. Op. cit.

[109] Smith, Jeffrey M. *Genetic Roulette,* 2007. Op cit. Pgs. 98-99.

[110] Corn Allergy. *Allergist.* Sponsored by the American College of Allergy, Asthma, & Immunology. www.acaai.org/allergist/allergies/Types/food-allergies/types/Pages/corn-allergy.aspx.

[111] Corn Allergy. FoodIntol. The Food Intolerance Institute of Australia. January 26, 2013. http://www.foodintol.com/corn-allergy.

[112] Corn Allergy Symptoms. *Livestrong,* Sept. 10, 2010. http://www.livestrong.com/article/250467-corn-allergy-symptoms/.

[113] Shetterly, Caitlin. The Bad Seed: The Health Risks of Genetically Modified Corn. *Elle,* August 2013, pp. 190-191, 246.

[114] U.S. Food and Drug Administration. Consumer Update: FDA Targets Trans Fat in Processed Foods. Nov. 7, 2013. http://www.fda.gov/forconsumers/consumerupdates/ucm372915.htm.

[115] Schmidt LA. New Unsweetened Truths about Sugar. *JAMA Internal Medicine.* 2014 Feb 3. doi: 10.1001/jamainternmed.2013.12991.

Chapter 4

[116] The American Academy of Environmental Medicine Calls for Immediate Moratorium on Genetically Modified Foods. *American Academy of Environmental Medicine* (press release), May 19, 2009. http://www.aaemonline.org/gmopressrelease.html.

[117] Genetically Modified Foods. *American Academy of Environmental Medicine.* Op cit.

[118] Seralini, GE, E Clair, R Mesnage, et al. Long Term Toxicity of a Roundup Herbicide and a Roundup-tolerant Genetically Modified Maize. *Food and Chemical Toxicity.* (2012), http://dx.doi.org/10.1016/j.fct.2012.08.005.

[119] *Genetic Roulette: The Gamble of Our Lives* [documentary], 2012, Op cit.

[120] Benbrook, Charles M. *Environmental Sciences Europe,* 2012, Op cit.

[121] Online Food Revolution Summit. Interview with Jeffrey Smith by John Robbins, April 28, 2013.

[122] Khan, Amir. Bee Colony Collapse Disorder Linked to Corn Insecticide. *International Business Times,* March 15, 2012. http://www.ibtimes.com/bee-colony-collapse-disorder-linked-corn-insecticide-425812.

[123] de Castilhos Ghisi N, and MM Cestari. Genotoxic Effects of the Herbicide Roundup in the Fish Corydoras paleatus (Jenyns 1842) After Short-Term, Environmentally Low Concentration Exposure. *Environmental Monitoring and Assessment,* 2013 Apr;185(4):3201-7. doi: 10.1007/s10661-012-2783-x. Epub 2012 Jul 22.

[124] King JJ, and RS Wagner. The Toxic Effects of Herbicide Roundup Regular on Pacific Northwestern Amphibians. *Northwestern Naturalist* 91(3):318-324. 2010 doi: http://dx.doi.org/10.1898/NWN09-25.1

[125] University of Pittsburgh. Even Small Doses of Popular Weed Killer Fatal to Frogs, Scientist Finds. *ScienceDaily,* 4 August 2005. http://www.sciencedaily.com/releases/2005/08/050804053212.htm.

[126] Schmidt Je, CU Braun, LP Whitehouse, et al. Effects of activated Bt transgene products (Cry1Ab, Cry3Bb) on immature stages of the ladybird Adalia bipunctata in laboatory ecotoxicity testing. *Archives of Environmental Contamination and Toxicology,* 2009 Feb;56(2):221-8. doi: 10.1007/s00244-008-9191-9. Epub 2008 Aug 20.

[127] Hilbeck A, JM McMillan, M Meier, et al. A Controversty Re-Visited: Is the coccinellid *Adalia bipunctata* Adversely Affected by Bt Toxins? *Environmental Sciences Europe,* 2012, 24:10 doi:10.1186/2190-4715-24-10.

[128] GM Watch. Monsanto: a history. http://www.gmwatch.org/gm-firms/10595-monsanto-a-history.

[129] GM Watch. The world's top 10 seed companies: Who owns nature? http://www.gmwatch.org/gm-firms/10558-the-worlds-top-ten-seed-companies-who-owns-nature.

[130] Online GMO Mini-Summit. Interview with Vandana Shiva by John Robbins, October 26, 2013.

Chapter 8
[131] Schmidt LA. New Unsweetened Truths about Sugar. *JAMA Internal Medicine.* 2014 Feb 3. doi: 10.1001/jamainternmed.2013.12991.

[132] Yang Q, Z Zhang, EW Gregg, et al. Added Sugar Intake and Cardiovascular Diseases Mortality among US Adults. *JAMA Internal Medicine.* 2014 Feb 3. doi: 10.1001/jamainternmed.2013.13563.

[133] Shaw RJ, and LC Cantley. Decoding Key Nodes in the Metabolism of Cancer Cells: Sugar and Spice and All Things Nice. *F1000 Biology Reports.* 2012;4:2. doi: 10.3410/B4-2. Epub 2012 Jan 3.

[134] *60 Minutes.* Is Sugar Toxic? April 1, 2012. http://www.cbsnews.com/videos/is-sugar-toxic/.

[135] Oyinlola Oyebode, Vanessa Gordon-Dseagu, Alice Walker, Jennifer S Mindell. Fruit and vegetable consumption and all-cause, cancer and CVD mortality: analysis of Health Survey for England data. *Journal of Epidemiology and Community Health,* 31 March 2014 doi: 10.1136/jech-2013-203500.

[136] Foley, Jonathan. It's time to rethink American's corn system. *Scientific American,* March 5, 2013. http://www.scientificamerican.com/article/time-to-rethink-corn/.

[137] Fallon, Sally, and Mary G. Enig. The Great Con-ola. *Weston A. Price Foundation,* July 28, 2002. http://www.westonaprice.org/health-topics/the-great-con-ola/.

[138] Chemicals in Our Food: What We Don't Know May Be Hurting Us. The Pew Charitable Trusts. April 9, 2013. http://www.pewhealth.org/other-resource/chemicals-in-our-food-what-we-dont-know-may-be-hurting-us-85899467015

[139] Online Food Revolution Summit. Interview with Michael Hansen, Ph.D., by John Robbins, April 28, 2014.

[140] Ibid.

[141] Emmott, Robin. Europe's Fear of GM Food and Meat from Cattle Raised with Growth Hormones Sows Divide. *Scientific American,* March 12, 2014. http://www.scientificamerican.com/article/europes-fear-of-gm-food-and-meat-from-cattle-raised-with-growth-hormones-sows-divide/.

Chapter 10

[142] Bloomberg News. Bayer Settles With Farmers Over Modified Rice Seeds. NYTimes.com. *The New York Times,* 1 July 2011. http://www.nytimes.com/2011/07/02/business/02rice.html.

[143] Organic Rice companies Impacted by GM Rice Contamination. *The Organic & Non-GMO Report,* November 2006. http://www.non-gmoreport. com/articles/nov06/gm_rice_contamination.php.

[144] Sabate, J. Nut Consumption and Body Weight. *American Journal of Clinical Nutrition,* 2003; 78(3 Suppl): 647S-650S.

[145] Non-GMO Project Standard. *Non-GMO Project,* June 2013. pp. 34-35. http://www.nongmoproject.org/wp-content/uploads/2013/06/Non-GMO-Project-Standard-v10.pdf.

[146] USDA. Organic 101: Can GMOs Be Used in Organic Products? May 17, 2013. http://blogs.usda.gov/2013/05/17/organic-101-can-gmos-be-used-in-organic-products/.

[147] International Federation of Organic Agricultural Movements. Definition of Organic Agriculture. http://www.ifoam.org/en/organic-landmarks/definition-organic-agriculture.

[148] Poongothai, A, R Ravikrishnan, and P Murthy. *Endocrine Disruption and Perspective Human Health Implications: A Review. The Internet Journal of Toxicology.* 2007 Volume 4 Number 2.

[149] Alavanja MC, JA Hoppin, and F Kamel. Health Effects of Chronic Pesticide Exposure: Cancer and Neurotoxicity. *Annual Review of Public Health.* 2004;25:155-97.

[150] Crinnion, WJ. Organic Foods Contain Higher Levels of Certain Nutrients, Lower Levels of Pesticides, and May Provide Health Benefits for the Consumer. *Alternative Medicine Review,* April 2010;15(1):4-12. http://www.altmedrev.com/publications/15/1/4.pdf.

[151] Benbrook CM, G Butler, MA Latif, et al. Organic Production Enhances Milk Nutritional Quality by Shifting Fatty Acid Composition: A United States-Wide, 18-Month Study. *PLoS ONE,* 2013; 8(12): e82429. doi:10.1371/journal.pone.0082429.

[152] Gallo, AC. Our Meat: No Antibiotics, Ever. *Whole Foods Market* (blog), June 25, 2012. http://www.wholefoodsmarket.com/blog/whole-story/our-meat-no-antibiotics-ever-0.

[153] Our Quality Standards: Unacceptable Ingredients for Food. *Whole Foods Market.* http://www.wholefoodsmarket.com/about-our-products/quality-standards/unacceptable-ingredients-food.

[154] Robinson, Jo. Grass-Fed Basics. *Eat Wild: The #1 Site for Grass-fed Food & Facts.* http://www.eatwild.com/basics.html.

[155] Daley CA, A Abbott, PS Doyle, et al. A review of the fatty acid profiles and antioxidant content in grass-fed and grain-fed beef. *Nutrition Journal* 2010, 9:10 doi:10.1186/1475-2891-9-10. http://www.nutritionj.com/content/9/1/10.

[156] Bailey, GD, BA Vanselow, et al. A study of the food borne pathogens: Campylobacter, Listeria and Yersinia, in faeces from slaughter-age cattle and sheep in Australia. *Communicable Diseases Intelligence,* 2003; 27(2): 249-57.

[157] Russell JB, F Diez-Gonzalez, and GN Jarvis. Potential Effect of Cattle Diets on the Transmission of Pathogenic Escherichia Coli to Humans. *Microbes and Infection 2,* 2000; no. 1: 45-53.

[158] Scott, Tony, T Klopfenstein, et al. Influence of Diet on Total and Acid Resistant E. coli and Colonic pH. *2000 Nebraska Beef Report,* pages 39-41.

[159] Robinson, Jo. *Why Grassfed is Best: The Surprising Benefits of Grassfed Meat, Eggs, and Dairy Products.* Vashon, WA: Vashon Island Press, 2000, pages 43-46.

[160] Information on GMO Sweet Corn. *Non-GMO Project.* http://www.nongmoproject.org/learn-more/sweetcorn/.

[161] GMOs at the Farmers Market. *Tracie Inman,* August 12, 2013. http://tracieinman.com/gmos-at-the-farmers-market/.

[162] Hu FB, and MJ Stampfer. Nut consumption and Risk of Coronary Heart Disease: A Review of Epidemiological Evidence. *Current Atherosclerosis Reports,* 1999 Nov;1(3):204-9.

[163] Fife, Bruce. *Cooking with Coconut Flour.* Colorado Springs, CO: Piccadilly Books, 2005.

[164] DebMandal M, and S Mandal. Coconut (Cocos nucifera L.: Arecaceae): in health promotion and disease prevention. *Asian Pacific Journal of Tropical Medicine,* 2011;4(3):241-247.

[165] Mercola, Joseph. Coconut Oil Benefits: When Fat is Good for You. *The Huffington Post,* February 14, 2011. http://www.huffingtonpost.com/dr-mercola/coconut-oil-benefits_b_821453.html.

[166] Fife, Bruce. *Cooking with Coconut Flour.* Op cit., p. 40.

[167] *The Dr. Oz Show.* Break Your Sugar Addiction, first broadcast on September 18, 2009.

Chapter 13

[168] AllergyKids Foundation. About Us page. http://www.allergykids.com/about-us/about-us/.

[169] Natural Resources Defense Council. Children, Cancer & The Environment. Q&A: Facts about Childhood Cancer. http://www.nrdc.org/health/kids/kidscancer/kidscancer5.asp.

[170] Le Beau, Christina. Boy meets Big Food: book review and giveaway. *Spoonfedblog* (blog), August 26, 2012. http://spoonfedblog.net/2012/08/26/boy-meets-big-food-book-review-and-giveaway/.

[171] Le Beau, Christina. About the blog. *Spoonfed* (blog). http://spoonfedblog.net/about/.

[172] Le Beau, Christina. Teaching your kids about food will not cause eating disorders. *Spoonfedblog* (blog), May 17, 2013. http://spoonfedblog.net/2013/05/17/teaching-your-kids-about-food-will-not-cause-eating-disorders/.

Chapter 14

[173] Peterson, Barbara H. Monsanto is Not 'Too Big to Fail' — Ban GMOs Now! *Farm Wars* (blog), October 1, 2013. http://farmwars.info/?p=11640.

[174] Rappoport, Jon. Are GMO Ballot Measures Just Another Covert Op? *Jon Rappoport's blog,* October 7, 2013. http://jonrappoport.wordpress.com/2013/10/07/are-gmo-ballot-measures-just-another-covert-op/.

[175] Local Voters Back GMO Ban in Big Numbers. *The Journal of the San Juan Islands,* November 7, 2012. http://www.sanjuanjournal.com/news/177740361.html.

[176] Koberstein, Paul. GMO companies are dousing Hawaiian island with toxic pesticides. *Grist,* June 16, 2014. http://grist.org/business-technology/gmo-companies-are-dousing-hawaiian-island-with-toxic-pesticides/.

[177] Mayor Kenoi Signs Bill 113. *Office of Mayor Billy Kenoi* (news release). December 5, 2013. http://hawaiicountymayor.com/2013/12/05/mayor-kenoi-signs-bill-113/.

[178] Koretz, Paul, O'Farrell, Mitch. Motion to the City of Los Angeles. Filed October 18, 2013. http://clkrep.lacity.org/onlinedocs/2013/13-1374_mot_10-18-13.pdf.

[179] GMO ban passes in Josephine, Jackson counties. KGW.com, May 20, 2014. http://www.kgw.com/story/local/2014/08/21/12638030/.

[180] Hofschneider, Anita. Maui Initiative to Ban GMO Crops Gets Enough Signatures for Ballot. *Honolulu Civil Beat,* June 6, 2014. http://www. civilbeat.com/2014/06/maui-initiative-to-ban-gmo-crops-gets-enough-signatures-for-ballot/,

[181] Yes on P 2014. About Measure P. http://yesonp2014.org/about-the-ordinance/.

[182] Walsh, Jim. A Secret Trade Deal is Threatening Our Safety. *Food & Water Watch* (blog), March 11, 2014. http://www.foodandwaterwatch.org/blogs/a-secret-trade-deal-is-threatening-our-safety/.

[183] Center for Food Safety Report Warns TTIP Could Undermine Critical Food Safety and Environmental Regulations. *Center for Food Safety* (press release), May 14, 2014. http://www.centerforfoodsafety.org/press-releases/3153/center-for-food-safety-report-warns-ttip-could-undermine-critical-food-safety-and-environmental-regulations.

Index

CPSIA information can be obtained
at www.ICGtesting.com
Printed in the USA
FSOW03n0059070916
24626FS